RELIEF FROM SOCIAL ANXIETY AND STRESS FOR TEENS

OVERCOME ANXIETY AND STRESS WITH CBT AND DBT SKILLS TO INCREASE MINDFULNESS AND COMMUNICATE SUCCESSFULLY

SUCCEED NOW

CONTENTS

INTRODUCTION

> " *It takes courage to grow up and become who you really are.*"

— E. E. CUMMINGS

Social anxiety always seems to arrive at the worst possible moment. You may be attending a party, heading to your classroom, or meeting someone new when suddenly, you are overwhelmed by the sensation that you are about to do something awkward or strange in public. Your palms start to sweat, you're sure you're blushing, and you are petrified of saying the wrong thing. It feels like nothing anyone could say could make it better, and even when friends or loved ones are around you, your symptoms can be just as intense. In fact, the more others tell you "there's nothing to worry about," the more utterly alone you may feel, and the more your fears may seem to be drowning you.

The following information may open your eyes to one important fact—anxiety is far more common than you may realize:[1]

- The National Institutes of Health reports that almost one in three people aged thirteen to eighteen will experience an anxiety disorder.
- Around 38 percent of female teens have anxiety, compared to 26.1 percent of males.
- Some 59 percent of teens find that balancing too many activities causes them to feel stressed.
- Around 37 percent of people say that stress makes them feel overwhelmed, 40 percent say it makes them irritable, while 30 percent claim it makes them feel sad or depressed.
- Social anxiety disorder (SAD) affects one out of three teens aged thirteen to eighteen.

FAQ: WHAT IS SOCIAL ANXIETY DISORDER?

People usually group many different types of disorder under the term "anxiety" in fact, there are five major types of anxiety disorder:[2]

- **Generalized Anxiety Disorder** (which is characterized by chronic anxiety and severe worry and tension).
- **Obsessive-Compulsive Disorder** (which often results in recurrent obsessions and repetitive behaviors).
- **Panic Disorder** (in which a person can have episodes of intense fear accompanied by physical symptoms like heart palpitations, chest pain, dizziness, abdominal issues, and shortness of breath).
- **Post-Traumatic Stress Disorders** (which can recur after exposure to a traumatic event such as military combat).
- **Social Anxiety Disorder** (which involves extreme self-consciousness or symptoms of anxiety in everyday social situations. Sometimes, fears are very specific (for instance, you may dread speaking in public or eating in front of others). At other times, they may creep up on you every time you are in a social setting).

Social Anxiety Disorder (SAD) is actually the most common anxiety disorder and the third most common mental health disorder in the US. If you have SAD, you may avoid new social situations, fear being judged in everyday social interactions, or worry intensely about upcoming social events.

Throughout this book, we will delve more into the nature and effects of SAD and anxiety as a whole. For now, it is simply important to know how far-reaching these disorders are, and to be aware of the fact that many people have more than one type of anxiety. For instance, you might have SAD but also occasionally have a panic attack, or you may have panic attacks without having Generalized Anxiety Disorder.

CELEBRITIES WHO BATTLE ANXIETY

When you think of Ryan Reynolds, Ariana Grande, or Taylor Swift, words like "confident," "charismatic" and "extroverted" probably spring to mind. However, all these big celebrities, who are called upon to bring their best smiles and panache to the red carpet, have wrestled with anxiety for years. Arian Grande, for instance, has PTSD, and she has said in the past that even her "anxiety has anxiety." She has quoted her idol, Jim Carrey (who has depression) many times, and once wrote the following Instagram post: "Performing is HELL."

Ryan Reynolds, the Deadpool actor who is a favorite on social media and is well-loved by audiences of all ages, recently opened up to a journalist from CBS, admitting that he has had anxiety his whole life.[3] He said, "I feel like I have two parts of my personality, that one takes over when that happens." He recalls having felt "overwhelmingly nervous" before appearing on a talk show. In the seconds before walking out before an audience, he would feel that he "would literally die" or that "something horrible would happen." As soon as the curtain opened, however, his calm self would take over and his heart and breathing rate would slow down, letting him know he would be okay. Getting to this precise moment, when you understand that you are in control and that you aren't actually in danger, is what we hope to help you achieve by the time you have finished reading this book.

Succeed Now is a network of like-minded individuals joined by a single mission: to offer our support and expertise to teenagers and young adults who are burdened by anxiety. All of us have spent decades studying Psychology, and many of us have helped teens with issues like social anxiety and depression. Throughout this book, we will be presenting true stories of adolescents we have taught or advised. You may find you can strongly relate to their struggles and experiences. We hope that you are motivated by the way many teens before you have managed to conquer anxiety so they could confidently do all the things they love.

Being the captain of your own ship begins with being aware of what anxiety is and how it can trick you into thinking you are in a situation of danger when you really aren't. It also involves recognizing your emotions, knowing how your personality can affect the way you view a situation, exercising emotional regulation, and taking part in specific exercises that can bring your stress levels down when you are presented with challenging situations.

By the time you finish reading this book, you will be familiar with cognitive-behavioral therapy (CBT) and dialectical behavior therapy (DBT). We will provide you with effective, practical exercises based on these therapies. You will learn useful shortcuts that can help you identify the presence of anxiety early, so you can nip it in the bud. As you try these exercises out, you will soon feel more confident and in command. You will realize that anxiety in itself is powerless when you take specific steps to end the "fight or flight response."

FAQ: WHAT ARE CBT AND DBT?

CBT and DBT are both considered "gold standard" treatments for social anxiety. Cognitive-behavioral therapy encourages you to understand the powerful link between how you think, feel, and behave. Its main goals are to change the negative thought patterns that can worsen emotional difficulties, and to encourage the adoption of healthy behaviors that can in turn have a positive effect on how you perceive a situation or person.

Dialectical behavior therapy is a type of cognitive-behavioral therapy. Its main aim is to help you live "in the moment," cope with stress healthily, regulate your emotions, and build positive relationships with others.

Throughout this book, we will be providing you with activities, exercises, and suggestions. Try them out, and study which of them produces the best results for you. Keep experimenting with the different strategies. Some will serve you well in specific situations; others may be the antidote you will be seeking in completely different circumstances. Some may not suit your personality or style, in which case you can simply let them go and consider getting back to them in the future.

Progress takes work, commitment, and a positive outlook. You may try one strategy and find that it instantly does the trick; another strategy may need a second or even a third go before it produces the desired result.

Throughout this book, we hope you perceive your progress from behind the lens of the "growth mentality." This viewpoint is opposite to that of a "fixed mindset." People with a fixed mindset believe that we are all born with fixed qualities (like intelligence and talent). They also believe that these qualities, rather than effort, are what create success. People with a growth mindset, on the other hand, believe that abilities can be developed and honed via dedication and hard work. They love learning and see mistakes and "failures" as magnificent opportunities to build resilience and grow as a person. A positive mindset is the difference between giving up because "social anxiety is just too difficult to overcome," and embracing a productive struggle that ends up with you at the helm. Be patient and exercise self-kindness, being as compassionate and supportive to yourself as you would to your best friend or loved one. Above all, remember that when social anxiety hits, it's the one time that your gut instinct may have got it wrong. Instead of running from anxiety, you need to face it head-on and show it who's boss. We hope to teach you exactly how to do that.

USEFUL LINKS

Sometimes, anxiety, depression, and stress can be severe or long-standing. If you feel overwhelmed, know that there are many resources you can contact. We will provide just four below, but know that there may be more resources in your area that may be worth contacting.[4]

- **SAMHSA (The Substance Abuse and Mental Health Services Administration)**

800-985-5990

This organization has a Disaster Distress Helpline, which provides 24/7 crisis counseling every single day of the year. When you call, you will be attended by trained crisis counselors, who will listen to you without judgment.

- **National Suicide Prevention Lifeline**

800-273-8255

This network of local crisis centers provides free emotional support to people who are emotionally distressed and/or those experiencing a suicidal crisis, 24/7, 365 days a year.

- **The Travor Project**

1-866-488-7386

A suicide prevention hotline that is catered for the LGBTQIA+ community. It has counselors that understand the specific challenges that members of the community can face.

- **Crisis Text Line**

Text HOME to 741741 to obtain help with problems like anxiety, depression, eating disorders, emotional abuse, self-harm, suicide, loneliness, and more. This service is also available at all times.

I AM BEATING ANXIETY

> "*Anxiety isn't you. It's something moving through you. It can leave out of the same door it came in.*"
>
> — JAMES CLEAR

Imagine you were in the woods and suddenly, you saw a wild bear approach you. Your heart would probably start beating fast, and you would begin to take in shorter, faster breaths. Blood would rush to your major muscle groups, to enable you to do one of two things: run away, or (if there was no other choice) defend yourself against a possible attack. Your hearing would sharpen and your perception of pain would drop. This is called the "fight or flight response."[1]

As you can imagine, this response is pretty useful when you are in a situation of actual danger. When anxiety strikes, however, it is often invoked just as quickly and strongly... the only difference is, you aren't in the wild and your life isn't actually under threat. This is arguably the toughest thing about anxiety—it can seem like you are facing a terrifying situation at any time of the day. Your symptoms can be so intense that they can interfere with your ability to build and sustain relationships. The good news is that you can learn how to manage stress, slow down the fight or flight response, and be aware of what is actually happening to you. Simply knowing more about anxiety can help you take action and regain control.

SOCIAL ANXIETY AND THE AMYGDALA

The amygdala is the part of the brain that is responsible for your body's fight or flight response. Action in this zone triggers the avalanche of symptoms associated with intense anxiety. When you are in a stressful or fearful situation, your mental focus shifts to another part of the brain—the prefrontal cortex—whose job is to calm you down when no real danger is present.

Brain scans have shown that people with social anxiety have hyperactivity in the amygdala. Moreover, the prefrontal cortex amplifies the activity of the amygdala instead of relaxing it. People with social anxiety can be so scared of other people's reactions that their brains interpret regular social interchanges as legitimate threats. No amount of rational thinking can completely calm them down. As overwhelming as social anxiety may be, however, know that your brain can be reprogrammed to behave more rationally during social interactions.

COMMON SYMPTOMS OF SOCIAL ANXIETY

If you have social anxiety, you may:[2]

- Dread situations in which others may judge you negatively.
- Experience intense stress when you do "force yourself" to attend a social occasion.
- Worry about doing something that makes you seem awkward.
- Be afraid of talking to strangers.
- Avoid stating your opinion because of a fear of how others might react.
- Have physical symptoms such as sweating, blushing, shaking, or unsteady speech.
- Analyze and judge the things you said or did when you were in public.
- Fear that others will notice you have anxiety.

- Expect the very worst possible outcome from a social situation.
- Be more irritable than in the past.
- Find it hard to concentrate.
- Have frequent stomach aches or headaches.
- Find that your grades have dropped.
- Find it difficult to sleep.
- Refuse (or be reluctant) to go to school.

A Worrisome Statistic: One symptom of anxiety that should be considered serious enough to seek help, is substance abuse. Self-medicating is certainly not exclusively a teen problem. Some people turn to substances as a way to numb their pain, feel more relaxed in the presence of others, or alleviate stress or pain. However, this is a poor coping mechanism because substances cannot erase the cause of social anxiety. They cannot teach you how to keep your symptoms in check in the long-term, or reduce your stress hormone levels. They are a short-term solution that can affect your relationships and your progress at school or college. They can also stop you from achieving professional success when you are older.

Nowadays, with vaping being as widespread as it is, some teens are turning to vaping substances like cannabis. Substances and alcohol do not solve the problem of social anxiety. They only make you dependent and, when you depend on anything, it can erode your self-confidence. You may feel that you literally cannot cope without alcohol or substances to calm yourself down—when in fact, you can.

The Symptoms of Social Anxiety May Vary

The symptoms of social anxiety can change over time. They can become more severe or frequent when you are undergoing periods of stress—which is why taking daily steps to keep your stress levels down is essential. Avoiding social situations may soothe you in the short term, but in the long term, they can stop you from leading your best life.

For instance, at school, you may be called upon to work collaboratively with classmates. This can be very tough if you are placed into a group with people you are not close to, or if you are expected to share ideas and engage in debate. By tackling stress proactively and taking your cues from CBT and DBT, you can start doing all the things that your anxiety may have stopped you from doing in the past. By knowing yourself better and embracing positive change, you can look forward to so many new experiences. These include:

- Making new friends.
- Attending high school or college parties and interacting with kids you may have always wanted to spend more time with.
- Starting, maintaining, and ending conversations comfortably.
- Meeting someone you like and doing something fun like going to the movies or grabbing a cup of coffee together.
- Returning clothing items to a shop.
- Enjoying a meal with others.
- Speaking in public.
- Knowing how to effectively calm yourself down if anxiety hits.

WHAT CAUSES SOCIAL ANXIETY?

It is difficult to pinpoint the exact cause of social anxiety. Possible causes include:[3]

- Learned behaviors. Some people can develop social anxiety after experiencing an embarrassing, awkward, or painful social event. Research has also linked social anxiety to over-protective parenting. Parents who are anxious in social settings may increase their children's likelihood of having this disorder.

- Having an overactive amygdala. When your amygdala is "hijacked," it is difficult to react rationally to a perceived threat.
- Inherited traits. Anxiety disorders tend to run in families, but scientists are yet to unlock the reason. These traits could be linked to genetics, but they could also be related to learned behaviors.

WHAT FACTORS CAN INCREASE THE RISK OF DEVELOPING SOCIAL ANXIETY DISORDER?

Risk factors for SAD include:

- Having a family history of the disorder (having close family members with an anxiety disorder).
- Being shy or withdrawn in new situations.
- Being on the receiving end of negative behaviors such as bullying, insulting, shaming, criticizing, and ridiculing.
- Having experienced trauma or abuse.
- Having an appearance or condition that draws attention. For instance, someone who stutters may be more reluctant to participate in conversations because of a fear of others' reactions.

- Having new, difficult tasks that can trigger SAD for the first time. You may encounter social anxiety for the first time if you are called upon to take part on a public debate or give a speech.
- Experiencing the death or alienation of a parent.
- Maternal distress during pregnancy or infancy

ANXIETY DISORDERS CAN BECOME MORE SEVERE IN THE TEEN YEARS

Some teens have been battling SAD and other anxiety disorders since they were children. In general, symptoms can get much worse during adolescence. The teen years are a challenging time indeed. There are more pressures to succeed at school and at extracurricular activities such as sports.

One big source of stress that arises during adolescence is peer pressure—the influence that people within your social group can have on you. Peer pressure is usually discussed in a negative light, but it can also be positive. For instance, your friends may influence you to engage in charity work or inspire you to join their study group. They may share helpful advice, encourage you to do your best, model good behavior, and help you learn vital social norms. All these things can help you grow as a person.

WHEN IS PEER PRESSURE NEGATIVE?

The downside of peer pressure is that you may be encouraged by schoolmates or friends to drink, vape, or try drugs. A survey conducted in 2022 showed that around 51.64 percent of people who used drugs as teens said they began doing so between the ages of 15 and 17. Alcohol was the most frequently used substance among girls and boys, followed by cannabis, then (among girls) prescription opioids and (among boys) stimulants.[4] When asked why they tried substances in their teen years, their answers included curiosity, peer pressure, and escaping from stress. Some were looking for a way to cope with mental health problems.

Negative peer pressure worsens the symptoms of anxiety and depression. It can also lead to arguments with loved ones, distract you from your schoolwork, and influence you to make risky or unhealthy choices. It can make you unhappy with how you look and lead to changes in behavior, since conforming to the standards set by others can be an endless and cruel battle.

This time in life can feel very restrictive, because you may find yourself worrying excessively about whether your peers see you as incompetent or uncool. You may also worry about saying something embarrassing or fear that others will make fun of you. Finally, peer pressure can erode your self-esteem and self-confidence. When you do things you really don't want to, it can cause you to lose faith in yourself.[5]

THE LINK BETWEEN SOCIAL ANXIETY AND DEPRESSION

It isn't difficult to see how SAD can indirectly lead to depression. For instance, if you are constantly backing out of plans with friends at the last minute, saying no to the chance to meet new people, or avoiding family gatherings, it may cause you to feel isolated. You may be aware of the importance of having friends and social support, but your anxiety may always "win out," causing you to say no when you actually want to say yes. The situation may make you feel sad, ashamed, or inadequate. If social anxiety does lead to depression, it is important to address your SAD symptoms while also treating your depression. Social anxiety and depression can have similar symptoms. For instance, both can lead to social withdrawal, feelings of worthlessness or shame, and confusion.

THE TEEN YEARS CAN BE CHALLENGING

There are many reasons why being an adolescent can be particularly stressful.[6] In addition to peer pressure, you may also find that you clash more than you used to with your parents. This can happen even if you get along with them and love them, because this is a time in which peers begin to wield a powerful influence on your life. It is also the start of your quest for your own identity. It can be a hard time for parents, too, as they suddenly have to adapt to different personality traits their children may display in the interim between childhood and adulthood.

HORMONES AND TEEN MENTAL HEALTH

Adolescence is a time of major hormonal fluctuations.[7] During puberty, there is a big spike in sex, adrenal, and growth hormones. All these affect your mood, emotions, and impulses. Teens with unbalanced hormonal levels can have a higher risk of having mental health problems. Moreover, big fluctuations in sex hormone (estrogen and testosterone) levels can result in anxiety, confusion, social withdrawal, and reduced self-esteem. Hormonal imbalances can be caused by genetics, poor nutrition, chronic stress, and environmental factors.

It is easy to see how the choices you make (including the foods you eat, how much exercise you get, and the extent to which you make stress reduction a priority) can have a big influence on your happiness and wellbeing. Did you know that by taking part in regular physical activity, you can regulate testosterone levels, thereby lowering your chances of having anxiety? If you want to start leading a healthier lifestyle, don't worry. We've got it covered with a host of strategies for you to try out (in Chapter Eight).

BRAIN DEVELOPMENT IN ADOLESCENCE

Teens are known for showing impulsive behaviors— that is, they may do things without weighing the conse- quences of their actions and do things "in the spur of the moment." Impulsivity has its upside; if you think too long before deciding to jump into a pool, take part in a race, or volunteer when someone needs a favor, you may not get a lot done!

On the other hand, impulsivity can be dangerous. For instance, statistics indicate that teens end up in emer- gency rooms owing to accidents more often than adults or children do. One reason teens can be more impul- sive is that their brains are more sensitive to immediate rewards (for instance, eating the cookie now instead of waiting). This is because the part of their brain that processes emotions goes through major changes, making rewards seem more appealing.

Research has shown, for instance, that in experiments in which teens are asked to choose between receiving a smaller amount of money immediately or a larger amount in the future, they tend to choose the former.[8] Adults, whose brains have built important pathways that enable them to postpone the need for rewards, usually wait for the larger amount of money.

You can, however, train your brain to think about the consequences of your actions. For instance, you might tell yourself, "I really feel like giving swim training a miss and playing computer games with my friends after school. However, if I keep at it, I could get chosen for the first team and maybe even take part in important competitions one day."

PHYSICAL CHANGES IN ADOLESCENCE

Adolescence is a period characterized by a big change in appearance. Kids who advance at a different rate from their peers can be self-conscious and feel more anxious. Girls, for instance, may feel uncomfortable if they develop much earlier. Boys, on the other hand, may feel embarrassed if their voice doesn't deepen when their peers' voices do, or if they go into puberty later and therefore look younger than their classmates. Some people can develop body dysmorphic disorder. They can become so fixated on a perceived flaw that it can cause them great distress and interfere with their ability to get on with their tasks and get on with others.

IS THERE SUCH A THING AS "NORMAL ANXIETY?"

Everyone feels a little anxious, as life is sometimes pretty stressful. If you are into sports, you may feel anxious about how you'll do in the minutes before your next match. Even if you love singing and regularly rehearse with a vocal coach, you may still feel butterflies in your tummy before performing for an audience. Many students are also anxious before exams. Their palms may sweat, and their hands may start to shake.

As bad as anxiety can be, try to find meaning from even the toughest experiences. Your nervousness can be useful because it may help you focus all your thoughts on the task at hand. Usually, anxiety goes away once you start the activity you were worried about. You may find that you get increasingly better at calming your nerves before an important occasion. As the years go by, you may also come to accept these feelings and sensations as a normal part of life. Knowing that you can still do well (even when you are nervous) and that these feelings are passing, can all help you feel more resilient. Anxiety does not define you; you can choose how you deal with it and become more confident in your ability to do so.

WHEN IS IT TIME TO SEEK HELP?

Most people instinctively know when social anxiety, panic attacks and other types of anxiety become a problem. For instance, you may find that you are scared of going to school or to your part-time job, or that you fear leaving the home or catching public transport. You may worry obsessively about an upcoming party, fearing you will blush, say something silly, or show how nervous you are. You may start avoiding social situations, to the point that you hardly leave home.

For some people, especially those who are prone to panic attacks, anxiety can be so overwhelming that they end up in the ER. Some symptoms of anxiety mimic those of serious conditions, and they can be so severe that the person experiencing them can seek medical attention. When people tell their doctor that they are experiencing heart palpitations, dizziness, and a faint feeling, they are often given tests like an electrocardiogram, a chest X-ray and blood tests. If the problem is anxiety, the physician may give the patient a temporary treatment.

Some people with anxiety visit their doctor various times, only to be told one thing: "It's 'just' anxiety." Of course, there is nothing small or insignificant about undergoing severe chest pains or feeling like you are about to lose consciousness. Never feel embarrassed about getting help when you feel something is not right. See a mental health professional and get a diagnosis if you can. Start, if you wish, by telling a parent, school counselor, or your family doctor about your symptoms. Hiding the problem and trying to "battle it out" by yourself will do little good. Friends and close family members can all provide crucial support during the times that you most need it.

Elena's Story

Elena was a 19-year-old college student who left her family home for the first time to study in California. She was thrilled at the thought of renting an apartment with other students for the first time and surviving on her own. However, a few weeks after her move, she found herself worrying incessantly about how she would behave in public. She was worried that when she entered her lecture rooms, other students would judge her negatively or laugh at what she was wearing, or the things she said. She was afraid to make eye contact with other students she didn't know well or to follow a conversation when someone tried to get to know her.

She had always enjoyed parties and dreamed of attending college functions and events, but her anxiety caused her to stay home by herself more and more. She feared that if she stepped outside her apartment, she would faint, and she was scared that this would happen while she was alone or on public transport. Things got very intense when she broke up with her high school boyfriend. Her best friend and roommate, Yasmin, would accompany her to emergency when she would get into a panicky state. Elena tried to take every step possible to avoid anxiety, but the more she restricted her social life, the more severe her anxiety grew. She sought the help of a mental health professional, who was a big help during her first year and beyond. Sometimes, you simply can't tackle severe anxiety on your own. The severity, consistency, and length of your symptoms will be a clear guide that you need helpful professional guidance. Don't keep the problem to yourself.

BREATHING IS POWERFUL

Breathing is more than just a technique you can use to soothe anxiety. It actually plays a role in many of the symptoms you may be encountering in the first, place, especially if you have panic attacks. As mentioned, when you are in fight or flight mode, you start taking shorter, shallower breaths, breathing with your chest instead of your belly. When you do so, you exhale more carbon dioxide than is usual. This changes the pH levels in your blood and causes a small decrease in the amount of oxygen that is released to your brain. The result may be a feeling like you are about to faint. The good news is that you won't lose consciousness. Fainting occurs when your blood pressure drops. When you are in the midst of a panic attack, however, your blood pressure rises slightly.

The problem with panic attacks is that you often don't realize the changes in your breathing patterns until it is too late, when you are either hyperventilating, feeling dizzy, or trying to calm down as your heart races madly. Rapid, short chest breathing can lead to additional symptoms, including chest pain (because you are using your chest muscles much more intensely than you usually do), tingling in your extremities or your face, and a sensation of breathlessness.[9]

If poor breathing techniques can trigger these terrible symptoms, controlled breathing does the opposite. It literally nips panic in the bud, sometimes so quickly it is surprising. Controlled breathing hones in on the way you exhale, relaxing you profoundly. If you have a baby sibling around you, take a look, and you will notice that they utilize belly breathing, expanding their belly when they inhale air. Controlled breathing ensures you do not take in too much oxygen, and it relieves pressure from your chest muscles.

The Science of Breathing

Study after study has shown that controlled breathing reduces panic and anxiety. One study by researchers at Southern Methodist University showed that respiratory training could help people learn to breathe in a way that reverses hyperventilation, producing a therapeutic change in carbon dioxide.[10] When you engage in controlled breathing, you may notice how, in just a few seconds, your heart rate begins to slow down. As this occurs, you start to feel more in control. Soon, you are able to take big, deep breaths and concentrate on the movement of your belly. You can control panic in this simple yet mighty way.

Are You Ready to Try Belly Breathing?

There are many breathing techniques you can try out, but it is a good idea to start with a classic exercise like belly breathing. To do so, follow these steps:

1. Relax your chest by slowly exhaling a little air, making it a point to "loosen" your chest and shoulder muscles.

2. Place one hand on your chest and another on your belly.

3. Inhale through your nose, pushing your belly out to let the air in. Your hand positioned on your stomach will help ensure that your abdomen, rather than your chest, is doing the work. Inhale as much air as you can, without forcing yourself to go beyond a comfortable level. If you have rhinitis or another condition, you can use your mouth. Just try to take in a small amount of air rather than a big gulp.

4. Pause for a little while and exhale through your nose or mouth, feeling your belly become smaller again. Aim to lengthen the exhalation little by little. For instance, try to count four seconds, then five, then six, as you slowly breathe out.

5. Repeat this exercise for three to five minutes.

Fun Fact: Women are more likely to be chest breathers than men because their ribs are more oblique (angled downward) than men's. Consider it a healthy adaptation for dealing with pregnancy. When pregnant bellies get larger, the dome of the diaphragm is less able to descend, limiting lung expansion.[11] As we age, however, both women and men lose as much as seven degrees of obliquity in their ribs. This means that their

respiratory volume decreases. In other words, you may find that chest breathing is comfortable now that you are a teen, but by your 50s, you may switch to belly breathing. Regardless of how you usually breathe, belly breathing as an exercise is useful for countering anxiety for people of all ages. Because it allows you to take in a large volume of air, you can extend the time of exhalation, which is a powerful way to achieve a calmer state.

APPS THAT SOOTHE

There are many apps that are focused primarily on breathing. Apps like *Breathe, Calm,* and *Headspace* all provide excellent exercises that can help you calm down when you feel anxious. The *Breathe* app teaches you to literally "watch your breath." There are animations that signal when to inhale and exhale, and you can customize the length of each breath. It's a pretty fun tool you can use when you're traveling to school or when you have a few free minutes.

More Breathing Exercises to Try

There are many more techniques which can help quell anxiety.[12] These include:

- **Breath Focus:** This technique is similar to belly breathing, It involves focusing on the rise and fall of your abdomen, and focusing on particular words when you exhale. You might use words like "relaxed" or "safe." You can imagine the air you exhale as washing over you like a slow wave, and imagine that the air you exhale carries away negative energy.

- **Equal Breathing:** This technique involves inhaling and exhaling for the same amount of time. For instance, you can slowly count the numbers "one-two-three-four" as you inhale, and the same numbers when you exhale. Focus on how your lungs fill up and empty themselves of air.

- **Resonant Breathing:** This technique involves breathing in through your nose for six seconds and exhaling for the same amount of time, slowly. You can try this technique out for around 10 minutes if you are comfortable doing so.

- **Pranayamic Breathing:** This breathing technique stems from the practice of yoga. It involves carrying out multiple breathing variations, including equal breathing and exhaling for a long period of time. It can also include alternate nostril breathing and lion's breath.

- **Alternate Nostril Breathing:** Sit in a comfortable spot, straightening your spine and opening your chest. Place your left hand on your lap and close your right nostril with your thumb, breathing in through your left nostril to the count of four. Next, close your left nostril as well, taking a brief pause. Open your right nostril and breathe out to the count of six. Now breathe in through your right nostril to the count of four, close your right nostril, take a pause with both nostrils closed and start the cycle again.

Lion's Breath: This exercise focuses on exhaling with force. Start off by kneeling, crossing your ankles and sitting on the bottom of your feet. You can also sit crossed-leg if it is more comfortable. Inhale through your nose and exhale with your mouth, saying "ha" as you do so. When you exhale, open your mouth widely and stick your tongue out, stretching it down towards your chin. Focus your mind on your "third eye" (located in the middle of the forehead) while you exhale. Relax your facial muscles and repeat the exercise up to six times.

Fun Fact: Equal Breathing is taught intensively to Australian Special Forces soldiers to use during actual

combat encounters. For this reason, the technique is also called combat breathing.

WHICH TECHNIQUE IS RIGHT FOR YOU?

Complete the table below, rating each technique from one to five (with one as the lowest score and five as the highest). Once you have tried them all, it will be very clear which are the best at soothing your anxiety.

Technique	1	2	3	4	5
Belly Breathing					
Breath Focus					
Equal Breathing					
Resonant Breathing					
Pranayamic Breathing					
Alternate Nostril Breathing					

In this chapter, we discussed social anxiety—its causes, risk factors, and symptoms. We also learned the importance of breathing as a way to nip panic attacks in the bud and reduce the myriad of physical and mental symptoms that can arise when anxiety takes over.

Breathing is an essential technique to hone from the start because it allows you to regain control over aspects such as your heart rate, sometimes in just seconds. In Chapter Two, we will talk about mindfulness, discussing techniques that will help you stop negative thoughts in their tracks and reduce overthinking.

2

I AM IN THE PRESENT

> 66 *"Stress is caused by being 'here' but wanting to be 'there,' or being in the present but wanting to be in the future."*

> — ECKHART TOLLE

If you have social anxiety, then you know how quickly negative thoughts and beliefs can quickly lead you to an anxious, fearful state. These thoughts can be irrational and harmful. They can magnify your feelings in such a way that you feel that others will reject you or that you will embarrass yourself in social settings. In order to stop these thought patterns in their tracks, you need to identify self-destructive thoughts, challenge their accuracy, and replace them with more positive ones.[1] In this chapter, we will help you achieve these aims through mindfulness. We will also offer exercises that directly question and put an end to negative core beliefs.

COGNITIVE DISTORTIONS: DEALING WITH A REALITY "WARP"

People with social anxiety can engage in "cognitive distortions." These are biased perspectives or patterns that are irrational. They are so subtle that they can become a regular part of your day-to-day thought process without you being aware of them. They can be incredibly damaging and can lead to anxiety and depression if left unchecked. Cognitive distortions have the following qualities in common:[2]

- They are patterns of thought or belief.
- They are inaccurate, irrational, or exaggerated.
- They can cause you psychological harm.

All people have cognitive distortions at one point or another in their lives. What makes these distortions a problem is when the person experiencing them does not identify or correct them, or when the distortions happen so frequently that they affect one's self-esteem or self-confidence. Some people are more skilled than others at stopping distortions from taking over their thoughts. However, even if you have never tried doing so before, know that it is a skill that can be learned.

THE LINK BETWEEN SOCIAL ANXIETY DISORDER AND COGNITIVE DISTORTIONS

Research published in the *European Journal of Psychiatry* showed that people with Social Anxiety Disorder have more cognitive distortions than control groups.[3] In particular, SAD can affect your tendency to use mental filters, overgeneralize, and personalize matters in social situations.

COMMON COGNITIVE DISTORTIONS

If you have an interest in psychology, you may enjoy reading the work of academics like Aaron Beck and David Burns. They contributed greatly to the subject of cognitive distortions. Burns' *Feeling Good Handbook*[4] lists numerous cognitive distortions, of which there are many. It can help to know what they are, so you can be vigilant of them if they pop into your mind. They include:

1. **Engaging in all-or-nothing thinking.** If you engage in this type of thinking, you may see everything in extremes. A person or thing is either wonderful or

terrible, you are either great or lousy at something, incredibly smart or dim, competent or useless. In fact, most situations and human beings do not lie at such polarized extremes.

Examples of all-or-nothing thinking:

- "I am hopeless at English. I will never understand Shakespeare. I'm just dumb!"
- "Nobody likes me at school."
- "I got a C on the test. The teacher might as well have given me an F."

2. Overgeneralizing situations. Something may happen once, and you may believe that it says something general about you, instead of seeing that all people have good and bad days and that positive and negative experiences. Examples of overgeneralizing:

- "I got a C on my Science test today. I am terrible at Science, and I'll never be able to get an A. I'll never get into my college of choice."
- "Jude said he couldn't come over today. He probably doesn't like me and doesn't want to hang out together. I'll never ask him to come over again."

- "The teacher disagreed with my viewpoint today. She hates me and thinks I'm a bad student."

Closely related to overgeneralizing situations is jumping to conclusions. For instance, if your boyfriend breaks up with you, you may tell yourself, "There must be something wrong or gross about me. No one I like will ever want to be with me again."

3. **Using a mental filter.** Someone may compliment you frequently yet say one negative thing, and you may filter out all the good and focus on the bad. This may cause you to see your relationship as over, despite all the positive things you may bring to each other's lives. The flip side of using a negative mental filter is ignoring positive comments, giving them little importance, or disqualifying them. **Examples of negative mental filters:**

- "My best friend forgot my birthday. She obviously doesn't care about me."
- "Tim told me to chill out while we were discussing our favorite bands today. He obviously doesn't respect my opinion and sees me as irrational and over-sensitive."
- "Sydney suggested that I wear my hair loose today. She obviously thinks I looked awful."

Examples of disqualifying positive comments:

- "My boss said I worked hard today. She probably just said that because nobody else was available last-minute."
- "My teacher said I asked interesting questions today. He was probably just being condescending."
- "Ewan said my hair was my best feature. It's probably because the rest of me is ugly."

4. Reading someone else's mind. People can be a true mystery and sometimes, we think we know what they are thinking or feeling when in fact, we can get it completely wrong. Examples of mind-reading:

- "Jen didn't say "Hi!" as effusively as she usually does. I think she's jealous because I've been hanging out more with Sofia."
- "Emma didn't answer my DM today. She's probably mad at me and couldn't be bothered telling me why."
- "Dina didn't "Like" my photo on Instagram. She probably thinks I look terrible."

This distortion is closely related to that of personalization because it involves applying a negative interpretation to a situation you may not know enough about. For instance, a friend may be moody because they've had an argument with a parent. When they're not their usual happy self at school, you may blame yourself or think they no longer like you.

5. Emotional reasoning. This distortion occurs when you take something you feel or believe as fact. For instance, you may feel like your best friend no longer likes you and prefers to hang out with other people, but this doesn't make it true. Examples of emotional reasoning:

- "I feel guilty, so I must have done something wrong."
- "I feel afraid, so the situation must be dangerous."
- "I don't feel good about myself, so I must be worthless."

6. Using "should" statements. While it is okay to remind yourself of important tasks or goals, watch for signs you are telling yourself what you "should" be doing too often. You may be setting too many rules for yourself, or setting the bar too high. When you are unable to comply with these rules, your self-esteem and self-confidence may suffer, which will only lead to more negative judgments about yourself. Examples of "should" statements:

- "I should be a better student."
- I should be smarter."
- I should be more fun."

7. Believing in fallacies of control, fairness, and change.

You may think that you have zero control of your life, or, on the contrary, feel that you are in complete control of everything (and therefore responsible for all the bad things that occur to yourself or others).

You may also judge your experiences through the lens of "fairness." If you think that something is unfair, it may hurt you deeply, and you may build up resentment, anger, and frustration. As hard as it is to accept, things aren't always logical or fair. Sometimes, even when you work hard for a goal, you may not achieve it. Instead of getting angry about the injustice of it all, try to grow from your experiences and obtain meaning from them.

A third common fallacy is that of change. You may believe that you can change someone if you "work on them" enough. In fact, nobody changes unless they want to. Moreover, pressuring someone to change to fit your ideals can result in greater resistance and in the continuance or worsening of behaviors you don't like.

8. Having to be right. If you interact with others on Twitter or other social media, you may notice people engage in huge debates and wars, metaphorically "fighting it to the death" because they have to "be right" or "win." Most of these arguments can be settled by simply accepting that people can have different opinions.

9. Personalizing things. You may blame yourself for circumstances that are not your fault, or you may assume you have been intentionally targeted or excluded. For instance, a friend from school may have a small dinner party and invite everyone from their dance class only. However, when you find out you are not invited, you may think it is because the host does not like you.

If you walk into a room and everyone stops talking, you may assume they are talking about you. If you have a family member who is struggling, you may blame yourself for not having tried hard enough or done better to help them out. It can be hard to comprehend that things are often simply beyond your control. It can also be challenging to rationalize events and comprehend that people sometimes make decisions because they are beyond their control. Their wish is not necessarily to slight or offend you. Try to give them the benefit of the doubt and to exercise empathy, so that the things they say or do don't hurt you so much.

Personalizing things causes you to feel responsible for others' happiness and their pain. It can also make you blame others when you are unhappy instead of making the positive changes you need.

WHY DO WE ENGAGE IN NEGATIVE THINKING AND COGNITIVE DISTORTIONS?

Most of us get into a cycle of negative thinking at some point in our lives. Psychologists sometimes refer to this type of thinking as "rumination." They believe that we engage in this activity in response to our anxieties about certain situations. Sometimes, we overthink things because we want to find a solution to our problems. However, rumination can have the opposite effect. Cognitive distortions destroy our ability to see our reality more clearly, and they can lead to anxiety, depression, and a sense of helplessness.

How Can You Put an End to Cognitive Distortions and Negative Thinking?

Dismantling cognitive distortions begins by being aware of them[5] and by being cognizant of the many harmful filters we can use throughout the day. If we frame our experiences more positively, avoid judgement and stop ourselves from jumping to the very worst possible conclusion, we can experience far less anxiety, and we can look forward to interactions with others.

SELF-ESTEEM AND SELF-CONFIDENCE: WHAT'S THE DIFFERENCE?

Throughout the book, we have often mentioned the words "self-esteem" and "self-confidence." These concepts play an important role in how you interact with others. From the outset, knowing the difference between the two is essential. Self-confidence is focused on abilities. For instance, you may feel confident about your piano playing, ability to write an essay, or talent at creating cool graphic designs.

Self-esteem is all about how you feel about yourself and how you value yourself. It is inward-facing, and it influences the way you relate with others.

Your self-esteem is shaped by many things, including your early childhood experiences, your family patterns, and the people who have played a vital role in your life. As such, people who have received heavy doses of criticism, shame, judgment, and other negative behaviors, can have poor self-esteem. This may exacerbate social anxiety and make them feel like they cannot change, grow, and build healthy relationships. Additional reasons for low self-esteem include being the victim of bullying or teasing, being ridiculed by schoolmates or friends, having others impose unrealistic standards on you, being neglected, and being abused physically, emotionally, or sexually.[6]

THE HURTFUL MESSAGES YOU CAN GIVE YOURSELF

Low self-esteem also leads to the cognitive distortion of mental filtering: absorbing the bad, and ignoring the good about yourself. It leads to negative messages such as "I'm just no good at socializing." "People just don't like me." "I'm not smart or funny enough to ever be popular." All these messages can stop someone with social anxiety from accepting an invitation, being calm in a social setting, or feeling confident about sharing their thoughts, feelings, and experiences with others. They can also make you fear "getting things wrong." If you feel you didn't do as well as you wanted in a social setting, it can cause radical behaviors such as refusing all future invitations.

SELF-ESTEEM AND PERFECTIONISM

People who have low self-esteem often set up rigid rules for themselves as a way to stay "safe." They may base all their value on something they are good at—for instance, school grades. For instance, you may tell yourself, "I have to get the highest grades on all English tests." If someone else gets a higher grade, you may tell yourself that you are hopeless, that there is nothing special about you, or that you are a "failure." Setting and working towards goals is great, but basing your self-esteem on achievements can be incredibly harmful. Be careful about setting rigid or unrealistic rules for yourself, as they can sap all your energy and stop you from enjoying balance in your life.

Psychologists often say that having a happy, satisfying life is about having many metaphoric "bottles" and ensuring that each is relatively full. If the bottle that represents your academic life is full to the brim, but other bottles are empty, why not try investing a little energy in filling the others up?

REFRAMING NEGATIVE BELIEFS ABOUT YOURSELF: A PRACTICAL EXERCISE

When you have an important goal such as overcoming social anxiety, keeping a journal is vital. Writing down your thoughts and emotions daily can help you identify negative thought patterns and beliefs, discover cognitive distortions, and see how poor self-esteem may be leading you to send yourself negative messages. To reframe your negative beliefs, take part in the following written exercise:

1. List down a few negative beliefs you may have about yourself. These can include:

- "Nobody wants to be my friend."
- "I have nothing interesting to talk about with others."
- "No one else has the same interests."
- "They think I'm uncool."
- "I'm not smart enough."

2. Reframe the statements with any evidence that is contrary to a negative message. For instance, you might transform the above statements in the following way:

- "Lisa and Tara are my friends."
- "I am a big Marvel fan and know all about many comic series. If I spoke a bit about this hobby, others might enjoy it."
- "There are millions of COD fans out there. Some of my classmates may enjoy playing."

- "I read a non-fiction book I really enjoyed. I might go to the bookstore or log onto Amazon to find more books that can enrich my vocabulary and help with my written work."

Your reframed statements should be based on real evidence, so they feel authentic to you. They should focus on the progress you are making (or the steps you are taking to achieve positive growth) instead of the results. For instance, if you are new to town, it's unrealistic to say, "I've made loads of good friends" but very positive to say, "I might sign up for the outdoor yoga class for teens. I am sure I will meet other kids who might go to the same school I will."

3. Ask yourself if you need more evidence to interpret a situation. In the example given above about your friend who threw a small dinner party, you may lack evidence as to why they did so. In time, a casual conversation may bring up the real reasons, but even if you never find out, it is important to know that people do things for many reasons, most of which you may not be aware of.

4. Ask what a friend would think about the situation. Would they give the situation a more positive spin? Would they make a joke about it and move on? Or would they also think it was pretty serious?

5. Ask how truly important the situation is to your life. Will it matter or be relevant a year from now or five years from now?

STRATEGIES FOR IMPROVING YOUR SELF-ESTEEM

In addition to reframing negative thoughts and messages, there are so many things you can do to feel happy with who you are. They include:

- **Challenge your self-critic.** Be fully in tune with the messages that are running through your mind. Be ready to "catch" thoughts like "I am no good at…" "I can't…" "Nobody…" and try to step back from the situation, viewing it before it makes its way through a negative filter.
- **Embrace the quality of empathy.** The people around you may not be their best selves on a given day. Instead of personalizing their behavior, understand that they may have things going on in their lives. When you have the chance to enjoy a quiet moment, ask them how things are going and if they are undergoing a difficult situation, let them know you are there to help.

- **Find healthy pastimes.** If you have gone through a problem over and over in your head, then you know that just staying home and having no outlet for your pain or stress, can be so frustrating it can get you in a slump. Think about taking a walk to a beautiful green or blue setting. Did you know that going to a park or being in a natural area for just 10 minutes reduces levels of the stress hormone, cortisol, in a powerful way?

When choosing a pastime, go with the things you love. If you adore dance music, then why not sign up for a spin class? If weights are your thing, why not join others in a communal CrossFit box? If nothing ignites your passion like cooking for others, why not try making gourmet meals or making a TikTok recipe? Everyone needs a healthy "escape" and when you're doing something you love, it's much easier to be "in the moment."

MINDFULNESS: LEARNING TO LET GO

You may have encountered the subject of mindfulness (the human ability to be fully present) in your learning or on the different social media apps you use. Mindfulness is a bit of a buzzword in the current health sector, but its benefits have been known for years. If you are scientifically curious, check out the many online studies on mindfulness and their benefits. There are so many studies on teens alone. Below are just a few fascinating findings:

- Secondary students who took part in an in-class mindfulness program enjoyed reductions in anxiety and depression up to six months later.[7]
- Mindfulness, combined with art, helps reduce stress-related headaches in teen girls.[8]
- Mindfulness meditation increases well-being in adolescent boys because it boosts their awareness of their ongoing experiences. The study showed that teens who had high levels of anxiety were the ones who benefited the most from mindfulness training.[9]

Additional benefits of mindfulness include decreased depression, better memory, cognitive improvements, enhanced relationships, improved decision-making, and better physical health.

New studies are constantly being published that expand the known benefits of mindfulness practice. One paper in 2022 found, for instance, that mindfulness meditation reduces pain by enabling people to "separate from the self."[10] That is, you can learn to experience thoughts and sensations while separating your sense of self from them. The study found that you don't have to be an expert to enjoy these effects. The findings hold great promise for looking for a fast-acting alternative to pain relief.

Mindfulness vs Mindfulness Meditation

Mindfulness and mindfulness meditation are sometimes confused with each other. Mindfulness involves achieving an awareness that arises from purposely paying attention in the present moment in a non-judgmental manner. You may recognize that you are currently tense, angry, sad, happy, or excited, without judging yourself for feeling one way or another. You simply acknowledge these emotions exist, without trying to repress them. By the same token, you don't allow them to "take over" or lead you to behaviors you may regret. When you are in the present moment, you acknowledge it is temporary. Your thoughts and emotions do not define you. That is, you may be angry in one moment because someone is late, but this does not make you an "angry person." You may be sad because someone was unkind to you, but this does not convert you into a "sad person." Through mindfulness and mindfulness meditation, you can learn to "ride" emotions like a wave, eventually moving to a state of calmness.

Mindfulness meditation is a mental training practice that focuses on slowing down racing thoughts, releasing negativity, and accepting your thoughts and feelings without judgment. It often involves deep breathing and focuses on sharpening your awareness of your body and mind. Mindfulness meditation is used in a wide array of settings. It can help people who are battling serious diseases like cancer or those who are grieving the loss of a loved one, owing to its powerful ability to reduce stress hormones. It is also used as a complementary therapy for substance abuse recovery. Consider mindfulness practice as one of the most effective tools you can use against panic attacks and anxiety.

A MINDFULNESS MEDITATION EXERCISE

You will find many useful resources that will help you hone mindfulness. I mentioned the apps *Calm* and *Headspace*, which have a host of excellent exercises targeting aspects such as stress, anxiety, focus, and sleep. You can start out with the following simple exercises for 10–15 minutes:

1. Find a peaceful spot at home; one that is quiet and all your own during your practice of meditation.

2. Wear something comfortable and sit on the floor or on a chair. Choose a comfortable position, keeping your body straight but not rigid.

3. Practice the belly breathing exercise we provided in Chapter One.

4. Notice your thoughts and emotions, accepting them as they are while focusing on your breathing.

5. Allow yourself to "not get it right the first time." You may find that negative thoughts or worries take over. Try to get back to breathing, but know that you will get better at keeping your mind "in the spectacular now."

Practical Mindfulness Exercises to Try

Being truly aware of how your thoughts and sensations can lead to social anxiety is important not only when you are setting aside a time to meditate, but throughout the day as well. Try the following exercises at school, at work, or when you're out and about with friends or family.[11]

- **Mindful eating:** Whether you are enjoying a full meal or a snack, try to use all your senses to fully appreciate it. For instance, if you are eating a kiwi fruit, hold it in your hands, feel its furry texture, peel it and smell its beautiful freshness. When you bite into it, notice if it is juicy and sweet. Chew slowly and savor each bite!

- **Mindful walking:** Find a quiet spot, preferably in the presence of nature. Pay attention to how you keep your balance as you move forward in slow motion. Take note of how the rest of your body—your shoulders, arms, and knees, move in unison. Breathe in and out in rhythm with your steps. Try to keep your mind on this activity itself, bringing your mind back to the moment if necessary by moving in slow motion and by breathing.

- **Mindful word:** Choose one positive word that puts you in a calm mood. It might be "love," "calm," or "acceptance." Think of the word, say it to yourself in your mind, then say it as you inhale and exhale air.

There are so many more opportunities for you to exercise mindfulness. Any activity you enjoy can be even more impactful if you are aware of the extent to which it fulfills, entertains, or amuses you. Being mindful is especially important when you are undertaking any activity that requires concentration—including driving. By keeping your eyes on the road, being in tune to conditions on the road and other vehicles and pedestrians, you can avoid the perils of distracted driving. Now, here's a little food for thought: The National Safety Council reports that cell phone use while driving leads to 1.6 million car crashes every year. One out of every four accidents, meanwhile, is caused by texting and driving. [12]

In this chapter, we talked about cognitive distortions and negative core beliefs, highlighting how they can affect your self-esteem. People with social anxiety may feel like they can never conquer their fears, because distortions lead them to view the world through a filter that interprets things in a negative light. They can also have low self-esteem and believe negative things about themselves which are not fact-based. To gain control over your social anxiety, it is important to be aware of the negative messages you give yourself, reframe your negative beliefs by taking an evidence-based approach, and understand how damaging distortions like personalization can be.

Mindfulness and meditation will help you keep your thoughts in the present moment, so you can enjoy all the special things that make being with friends and loved ones so special—the sound of their laughter, the smells of home cooking, and the majestic natural surroundings you can enjoy together.

Now that you are aware of the things that can bring you down, it's time to build your resilience. In Chapter Three, we will discuss key strategies that can help you face challenges, build the social skills you need to overcome obstacles, and adopt positive thinking habits.

3

I AM RESILIENT

> " *"The human capacity for burden is like bamboo —far more flexible than you'd ever believe at first glance."*
>
> — JODI PICOULT

The teen years are often celebrated as some of the best in a person's life. However, shows like *Euphoria*, *Heartstoppers*, or *Stranger Things* reveal the tougher side to teen life. Peer pressure, the wish to be liked, and coping with negative experiences like teasing and bullying are tough, especially when you haven't gathered the experience you need to bounce back. Resilience—remaining strong in the face of setbacks— is crucial, not only because it helps you recover, but also because it helps you turn negative experiences into positive life lessons.

Think of the most resilient people you know and love. You may have a grandparent, parent, sibling, or friend who has been through big shifts in their life like losing a loved one, being fired from a job, or being let down by a friend or partner. Yet they may have grown from adversity, and they may often have many wise words to say about how to deal with disappointment. Hold onto wise words. Value the experiences of the people you love. They may not echo your own, but the strategies they used to bounce back can help you make it through an issue that is distressing you.

No one is resilient all the time. You may find that your own resilience can go up and down, and that you are better at recovering from some setbacks than from others.

EXAMPLES OF RESILIENCE

Resilience can consist of:

- Recovering after a painful or tough experience.
- Giving something a try, even if it didn't work out the way you wanted the first time around.

- Accepting the things you cannot change and working on the things you can change positively.
- Standing up for yourself.
- Looking for the good things you learned from a challenging circumstance.

Logan's Story

Logan was 13 years old when his parents told him they were getting a divorce. Although his mom and dad reassured him that they would still be a family and that he would spend equal time with both of them, he feared that life was changing too quickly. Logan sometimes blamed himself for his parents' breakup because they used to argue about aspects of his life (whether he should learn Chinese, what sport he should do, and where he should go to school).

In the beginning, it was particularly difficult because his parents were not getting along, and he found that he was acting as a messenger between them both. Sometimes they would argue, and he felt like both of them wanted him to take sides.

Logan's grades started slipping. Because of the tension he would feel when he was with his parents, he started spending more time at the gym and withdrawing from friends because he didn't know how to explain how he was feeling. Logan developed anxiety and began having panic attacks. When this happened, he stopped wanting to go to school and didn't pick the phone up, even when his best friend, Tristan called.

One day, he had a panic attack at school and his teacher suggested that he should talk to the school psychologist, Ms. Lawton. He told her that he felt he was to blame for the big shake-up that had occurred in his family. Miss Lawton suggested talking to his parents about how he was feeling. She also had a meeting with his parents a few days later. When they realized the extent to which the divorce was affecting their son's well-being, they did something that Logan never dreamed possible. They attended therapy to work as a parenting team more collaboratively. Logan also saw a specialist who helped him find solutions to challenges and who shed light on the fact that divorce may be painful to accept, but it does not mean you no longer have a family. Nor does it mean your parents do not love you. In time, Logan began to reach out to friends and explain what he was going through. He learned that some of his friends had been through the same anguish. Not all of them had parents who were able or willing to work collaboratively, or who could afford a specialist's help. However, everyone had interesting experiences and great advice on how they built their resilience during this difficult time.

THE ROLE OF RESILIENCE IN CURBING SOCIAL ANXIETY

People who are resilient have lower levels of social anxiety. One possible explanation is that people who are resilient tend to evaluate themselves positively, be confident in how they are performing, believe in their decisions, state their opinions more frequently, and have a low expectation of failure. Resilient people also tend to have good social skills, which enables them to communicate well with others. These skills enable them to react appropriately to others, which in turn reduces the chance of negative self-evaluation.[1]

THE IMPORTANCE OF RESILIENCE IN ONLINE INTERACTIONS

When you are resilient, you are more adept at facing challenges instead of avoiding them. Research by Penn State University researchers found that when it comes to online risks, it is better to boost resilience than to ban teens from using the Internet.[2] In their study, resilient adolescents were less likely to experience negative effects even if they were online more frequently. The researchers found that Internet exposure is not in itself a problem. It is okay to interact with others on social media, so long as you learn how to cope with the stress it can bring. You should also learn how to reduce your chances of being exposed to online risks by employing tried-and-tested cyber safety strategies.

For instance, if you are on your favorite app and a friend asks you for an intimate photo, you could succumb and send one if you didn't know the risks involved. If you build up your resistance, however, you can be more comfortable about saying no and reduce the risk of your private information being shared online.

THE SEVEN STEPS TO GREATER RESILIENCE

There are five main steps involved in being resilient. Working on each of them is important if you want to enjoy a good social life and feel comfortable in the company of others.

1. Be Kind to Yourself

When a friend is having a bad day, you probably look for ways to lift their spirits, let them know that you are there for them, and try to stop them from blaming or judging themselves. However, how often do you do these things for yourself when you are feeling anxious, stressed, or sad?

Self-compassion (being as kind to yourself as you would to someone you love) is a vital pillar of resilience. It enables you to see yourself as human and, therefore, fallible. One study published by academics at the Australian Catholic University found that self-kindness can help protect teens and adults alike from the harmful effects of perfectionism.[3] If you are a perfectionist, then you may be over-critical of yourself and exercise little patience when you make mistakes.[4]

To be more self-compassionate:

1. Allow yourself to make mistakes.
2. Care for yourself as you would others.
3. Let go of the need for validation from others.
4. Use self-compassion affirmations. These include statements like:

- "I can do this."
- "I can learn important lessons from my mistakes."
- "I'm going to be as generous with myself as I would with my best friend."

Writing a Self-Compassion Letter

If you enjoy writing, you might benefit from writing yourself a self-compassion letter. Use your journal to do so, writing to yourself as you would to a friend. Writing alleviates the worry, shame, sadness, and fear that can arise when you engage in negative thought cycles. In your letter, you can use phrases like:

- " I forgive myself for feeling as hurt as I did this morning..."
- "Every day is a new day. Today was not my last chance to exercise kindness and empathy..."
- "I behaved this way today because_____. Next time, I can try to make up for it by showing that I care/listening to my friend with my undivided attention/doing the favor Tristan asked me for..."

2. Sharpen Your Emotional Awareness

Anxiety can build up if you don't stop frequently throughout the day to think about how you're feeling. Painful emotions and sensations (such as feeling rejected or ignored, being anxious in a specific class at school, or being teased) can spark self-judgement and lead you to say negative messages to yourself. Try to build a moment-by-moment awareness of your emotions in a gentle, loving way. Take frequent pauses throughout the day to do the following:

- Engage in mindfulness practice by recognizing the emotions and thoughts you may be having. Label them and accept them.
- Recognize that these thoughts and emotions are temporary. They will pass.
- Try to understand the reasons why you are feeling the way you are.
- Free yourself from the need to control or repress these thoughts and emotions.

Use Plutchik's Wheel of Emotions

Sometimes, it can be hard to identify exactly how you are feeling. A great tool to have at hand in Plutchik's Wheel of Emotions, which identifies eight basic emotions:[5]

- Joy
- Trust
- Fear
- Surprise
- Sadness
- Disgust
- Anger
- Anticipation

Each emotion has various intensities. For instance, joy in a less intense state can be felt as serenity. In its most intense state, it can be called ecstasy. Anger in its lightest state can be called annoyance; in its strongest state, it is rage. Naming your emotions as precisely as possible is important because it gives you important information about the situations and experiences that cause you the most distress. With this information, you can take steps to reframe the situation in a more positive way, or set boundaries that will protect you in the future.

Once again, journaling your emotions and the situations that cause them can help you identify negative patterns that are getting you stuck in a rut. When you notice these patterns, you can list them down and try a few strategies that will enable you to break free of them.

3. Learn How to Set Boundaries

If you sometimes find it hard to say no, know that millions of people of all ages have this exact same difficulty. People with a high level of empathy, in particular, can find it devastating to let someone down. As difficult as it may be, saying no is an important part of setting your boundaries. If you accede to every request, do every favor you are asked for, and put your own health and wellbeing on the back burner, you could end up feeling fatigued, tired, and even angry—at yourself, more than anyone else.

Setting healthy boundaries helps you feel more comfortable in social settings because you never need to worry that someone will ask you to share information you are uncomfortable with, or do something that doesn't feel right.

Experience is the best teacher when it comes to boundary setting, but starting in your teen years will stand you in good stead for the rest of your life. It will help you feel more confident about going to parties, get-togethers, and school events, since through practice, you will learn how empowering it can feel to identify, share, and respect your own boundaries.

There Are Three Types of Boundaries:[6]

- **Emotional Boundaries:** These include talking about personal matters when you're ready, enjoying "me time" when you need to be alone, and allowing friends to be upset without having to "fix" their problems.
- **Physical Boundaries:** You have the right to your personal space and to greet and interact with people in a way you are comfortable with.
- **Online Boundaries:** You should decide what you feel comfortable about sharing online with others.

You should feel free to deny someone's request for your password and be able to say "no" if someone asks to see a personal device like your phone.

Setting boundaries is a vital way to build self-kindness and resilience. When you do so, avoid telling white lies or asking what you need in a roundabout way. Speak assertively, looking others in the eye with a straight and confident posture. Examples of assertive statements you might make to establish your personal limits include:

- "I would love to join you guys for a GTA match, but I'm going to CrossFit today."
- "I prefer to stand at this distance, if that is okay."
- "Sorry, I don't share my phone with anyone."

When in doubt, use the word "don't" instead of "can't." It will keep you safe from peer pressure because it is a clear assertion that you simply do not do something (not now, not ever). If someone insists on crossing your boundaries, assertively let them know that you have set your limits for a reason, and you always respect them. If a friend wants you "all to themselves," let them know that although they mean the world to you, other relationships are also important in your life.

Respect Your Own Boundaries

The easiest way to get others to respect your boundaries is to do the same. Do not give in to controlling behavior or manipulative phrases like "If you were my friend, you would do this." "Why are you so square?" or "You're so boring." If, for instance, you are unable to attend a social occasion and your friend tries to make you feel guilty, let them know that you understand they would like to go with you. However, explain that your upcoming exam is very important and that studying for it is non-negotiable. Be kind and use humor to diffuse tense situations, but don't back down or give in to ultimatums. Be around people who support your goals, believe in you, and make you feel great about succeeding.

Setting New Boundaries Can Be Challenging

If you have always said yes to friends, and you suddenly stop acceding to their demands, you may find resistance on their part. To some extent, this is to be expected, because patterns can be hard to break. Your friends may behave in a way that makes you feel guilty or scared of losing their friendship, all in an attempt to make things change back to how they used to be. Don't give up, stick to your resolve and eventually, they will understand that your boundaries are firm. During a calm moment, if they ask you why you have changed a few things, calmly explain that you are trying to build your resilience by setting boundaries that will make you more comfortable, confident, and happy.

4. Know Your Personality Traits

Teens in high school often idolize popular kids, thinking things like, "I wish I was as outgoing as Sandra," "I wish I could play football like Leo," or "I wish I was as confident as Tim." While admiring people can be motivating and can push you to be your best self, building resilience very much depends on knowing yourself well, accepting your personality type, and knowing your strengths and weaknesses. This does not mean you have to avoid working on aspects of your personality or behavior you want to improve. However, it does involve understanding that people are different. We each have things that make us special, as well as things we work on. You don't have to be like anybody else to have a happy, healthy social life. Of course, keeping an open mind, observing, and emulating positive behaviors are all intelligent courses of action.

How Many Personality Dimensions Are There?

After hundreds of years of study, academics are still debating as to exactly how many personality types there are. However, many agree that there are five big personality dimensions or traits, which most of us have to a greater or lesser extent.

The Five Main Personality Traits

The five basic dimensions of personality are:[7]

- **Extroversion:** This trait is characterized by talkativeness, assertiveness, and sociability. People who are extroverted tend to love starting conversations and being the center of attention. They have a big friend circle and find it easy to make new acquaintances and friends. Being around people boosts their energy. People with lower levels of extraversion may prefer being alone. Socializing with others can wrest from (rather than restore) their energy. They may not be much into small talk and do not enjoy being in the spotlight.
- **Agreeableness:** Trust, kindness, affection, and altruism are just a few attributes associated with this dimension. People with high levels of agreeableness care a lot about others and have a high degree of empathy. They enjoy helping

those in need. Those with lower levels of this trait have little interest in how others feel. They may insult, manipulate, or belittle others.

- **Openness:** This dimension includes imagination and insight. People with a high degree of openness tend to have a wide range of interests, and they go about life with a positive curiosity about the world and people. They love enjoying new experiences and are open to learning new things. Those who are low on this trait tend to be uncomfortable with change. They may dislike talking or learning about theoretical or abstract concepts.

- **Conscientiousness:** This trait is linked to good impulse control and the ability to work towards goals. Those who score high in this trait usually manage their time well and enjoy following a schedule. Those who rate low in this trait dislike structure and tend to procrastinate or fail to complete set tasks.

- **Neuroticism:** This dimension is characterized by emotional instability, sadness, and moodiness. Those who rate highly in neuroticism may experience stress, be anxious, or get upset easily. Those who are low in this trait are usually described by others as "stable" and they don't worry too much about things.

There are many free online resources, such as Truity's *The Big Five Personality Test,* which will enable you to learn a bit more about yourself.[8] By knowing your strengths and weaknesses, you can identify areas you may wish to work on. Obtaining a better understanding of the different dimensions that make up your personality also enables you to accept yourself. Each of us is different, and there is no "high score" or "low score" that can judge human beings as a whole.

Most People Lie Within a Spectrum of the Personality Dimensions

You may wish that you had more friends like your classmate, Jamil. He always seems to be surrounded by others and is typically the center of attention because of his great sense of humor and conversational skills. Jamil is someone you might describe as a true extrovert. However, recent research indicates that between one-half and two-thirds of people are actually ambiverts; that is, they have a balance of introverted and extroverted traits.[9] This can actually be a big advantage, with studies indicating that ambiverts are better salespeople than introverts or extroverts. The reason is that they are able to be assertive and chatty, or listen to others, depending on the circumstances. Some situations call for us to listen and reflect on the information we are receiving, while others require us to be charismatic and confident. As you grow in age and experience, you can learn to identify the type of situations that call for each type of behavior.

How Many Friends Do Average Teens Have?

The vast majority of teens in the US (78 percent) have between one and five close friends. Only 20 percent have six or more close friends. Around 87 percent of teens make close friends at school, and around 61 percent of close friends are of a different gender, 60 percent are of a different ethnicity, and 46 percent are of a different religion. Some 15 percent of close friends first meet online and 35 percent of friends live far away.[10] The statistics are food for thought, as they show that although teens can be surrounded by big groups, most are actually close to only a handful of people (or fewer). Therefore, if you have one or two good friends, you are very much part of the majority.

5. Keep Things in Perspective

Being realistic and thinking things through are vital if you wish to be more resilient against issues that can arise daily. For instance, it may seem like the end of the world if your best friend joins the school basketball team, and it means you won't be seeing as much of them. Find positive aspects to the situation. For instance, your friend may only train twice a week and still have a good amount of time to spend with you regularly. Moreover, you can enjoy watching them compete and achieve their dreams of becoming a professional player. When a problem arises, use your journal to answer the following questions:[11]

1. How bad is this, really, from one to ten?
2. Why is this a problem, or why is it causing me pain or distress?
3. What are a few possible solutions to this problem?
4. Which of these solutions seem the most interesting to try?
5. What practical steps will I take to put my chosen solution into action?

After trying out one or more solutions, write down how each worked out. Keep experimenting until you find the strategies that work best for you. Doing so will stand you in good stead, not only during your teen years, but also when you are an adult.

6. Treat Others Kindly

Treating friends kindly, listening to them when they need to talk to you, and being empathetic will all help maintain and strengthen the friendships you have. Talk show host Oprah Winfrey, once said, "Lots of people want to ride with you in the limo, but what you want is someone who will take the bus with you when the limo breaks down." However, friendship is about more than just being there when times are tough. It also involves sharing quality time, prioritizing one's friendship, and trying to make others happy.

Kindness and the Art of Active Listening

When a friend is sharing their ups and downs with you, listen to them actively, so they feel you really care about what they are saying. Active listening may also give you the chance to hear how they cope and perceive situations, and this can help you if you have social anxiety. Active listening techniques include:

1. Using open body language (keeping your arms to your sides and your palms facing the person, looking them in the eyes, and nodding occasionally to show you're on their wavelength).
2. Waiting for your friend to finish speaking before sharing your thoughts. People sometimes feel unheard if others interrupt them or start talking before they have fully finished their sentences.

3. Using phrases that show you understand. Simple phrases that work well include: "Oh, I see," "I understand," and "Yes, that does sound tough."

4. Being in tune with your friend's needs. Some friends simply need someone to listen to them; they don't necessarily want their friends to rush in and "fix things." Others do enjoy receiving advice. The best rule of thumb is to only offer advice when someone asks you for it. When doing so, be gentle but honest. It's easy to simply agree with everything friends say, but a good friend will speak from the heart and let their friend know how they think or feel about a situation.

7. Aim to Get Things Done

The more you achieve your goals, meet deadlines, and solve problems that come your way, the more resilient you are bound to be. In addition to setting a regular schedule for aspects like study, socialization, gaming, and sleep, consider pursuing any talents you wish to explore. For instance, if you have a beautiful voice, why not sign up for the school musical? Joining a school play involves commitment and consistency, and it is a great way to meet cool people you never knew shared the same interests as you. Taking part in a competition, forming part of a group that cleans up beaches and green areas, or signing up for mountain trekking are all activities that can boost your confidence and put you into contact with like-minded teens.

PRACTICAL EXERCISE: REFLECT ON YOUR RESILIENCE

Divide a page in your journal into various boxes. Within these boxes, list the times when you have been resilient and overcome obstacles. You can use text, drawings, or a combination of both Below, you will find a few examples of the type of subjects you might cover:

I was resilient when... I failed my math teast, but worked harder to study and passed it the next time I tried.	*I was resilient when...* My parents got divorced and I felt stuck in the middle, but was able to stay strong throughout and be myself no matter what.
I was resilient when... I got a lower grade than I expected after studying so hard. I talked to the teacher and asked how I could improve and will try her suggested strategies next time.	*I was resilient when...* I wasn't accepted into the track team, so I decided to sign up for swimming to build up my fitness level.
I am going to become more resilient by... Making sure I spent at least 30 mins each day doing something relaxing, such as meditating in my garden, cooking, or listening to music.	*I am going to become more resilient by...* Training hard, so I am accepted into the track team next time.
I am going to become more resilient by... Practicing my active listening techniques.	*I am going to become more resilient by...* Making it a point to sleep at least eight hours a night, so I feel strong and energetic the next day.

In this chapter, you may have discovered that being resilient isn't just a matter of "toughing it out" or holding your head high in the face of obstacles.

Resilience arises from a myriad of factors, some of which seem to have very little in common with each other. For instance, being kind to yourself enables you to avoid taking things personally or judging and blaming yourself when something negative happens. Working on your emotional awareness, meanwhile, allows you to be sensitive to how you are feeling and to take the steps you need to calm yourself down or take a break.

Setting boundaries is one of the most important skills resilient people rely on regularly. It is okay to say no without feeling embarrassed or fearful that people will no longer like you. They make poke fun at you or show disappointment if you don't accede to their demands, but in the long run, they will respect you.

We mentioned how personality can affect the way you enjoy interacting with others. People with social anxiety can sometimes feel like they "should" be more extroverted, have more friends, or enjoy the same activities everyone else is. Being true to yourself is a key aspect of resilience. Moreover, most people truly connect with just a few people. Their friends accept them as they are and do not force them to do things they are uncomfortable with.

Finally, build your strength up by keeping problems in perspective and realizing that most issues that worry you terribly today may be completely irrelevant in the future. Be kind to others along the way, for they will support you when you are undergoing difficulties. Aim to set and achieve goals, focusing on two main things: the effort you are investing in the attainment of your goal, and the importance of learning from mistakes.

When something doesn't turn out how you wanted, write down a few strategies you can try out next time, so you achieve outcomes you are happier with.

The next chapter is closely related to this one because it focuses on strengthening your mindset by believing in the power of change and growth. Most people who are successful have had to work very hard to attain their goals. Some (including soccer star Cristiano Ronaldo) faced big obstacles in their childhood – including poverty and a lack of opportunities. Even Ronaldo was once a beginner who had to learn how to kick a ball with the right technique. Who would have known that his first attempts at playing this challenging sport would mark the beginning of a spectacular career. In October 2022, Ronaldo achieved his 700th goal!

4

I HAVE A STRONG MINDSET

66 *"Always do what you are afraid to do."*

— RALPH WALDO EMERSON

In the Introduction, we spoke a little about the importance of facing challenges with a growth mindset. In this chapter, we will explain a little bit about how the brain works, delving into the subject of neuroplasticity and how it is compatible with a growth mindset. We will also suggest a series of positive affirmations you can use at home.

Fun Fact: Neurons are your brain's information messengers. They transmit information between different areas of the brain (and between the brain and

the rest of the nervous system) through electrical impulses and chemical signals. There are as many neurons in your brain as there are stars in the Milky Way (about 100 billion!).

YOUR BRAIN IS AWESOME

Think back to the first time you learned to ride a bike. Keeping your balance may have seemed close to impossible. You may have had to use training wheels until you felt more confident, then had someone run by your side until you felt confident you wouldn't fall. If you're like most kids, you probably did fall a couple of times. Of course, once you got a handle on it, cycling began to seem like second nature and to this day, you may wonder how you could have found it so difficult when you first started. When you come to think of it, your accomplishment is pretty impressive. It can be attributed to neuroplasticity—the science behind the growth mindset.[1]

THE DIFFERENT PARTS OF THE BRAIN

The brain has three main parts:[2]

- **The cerebrum.** This is the largest part of the brain, and it comprises right and left hemispheres. It is responsible for higher functions like seeing, hearing, speaking interpreting touch, reasoning, learning, and the emotions. It also performs fine movement control.

- **The cerebellum.** This is a much smaller structure nestled beneath the cerebrum. Its role is to coordinate muscle movements and maintain posture and balance.
- **The brainstem.** A relay center that connects the other parts of the brain to the spinal cord. It performs many automatic functions, including breathing, body temperature, the heart rate, wake and sleep cycles, swallowing, coughing, and sneezing.

There are other important parts in the brain that affect the way you think and feel. These include:

- **The prefrontal cortex.** This part of the brain is located just behind your forehead. It plays a central role in attention, impulse inhibition, and prospective memory (remembering to perform a planned action or intention in the future).[3]
- **The amygdala.** The amygdala plays a key role in detecting threats and activating the fight or

flight response. The amygdala can be found deep in the center of your brain.

- **The hippocampus.** This part of the brain plays a major role in learning and memory. It is located within the center of the brain.

WHAT ARE NEURONS AND PATHWAYS?

Neurons are tiny cells that send messages to each other. They produce electric signals to send messages to numerous cells in your body, telling them what to do. When you perform an action frequently enough, your brain makes a connection or pathway between neurons and the next time you perform the activity, it is easier. The brain is a little like a physical muscle in that the more you use it, the stronger it grows. Practicing the things you learn and continuously embracing new challenges are important ways to promote neuroplasticity.

WHAT IS NEUROPLASTICITY?

Neuroplasticity (or brain plasticity) is your brain's ability to grow and change throughout your lifetime. Until relatively recently, scientists through this ability was limited to childhood. They believed that the creation of new neurons stopped shortly after birth, and that the adult brain was stable and unchanging.

However, recent research has shown that the brain continues to change even in our senior years. In particular, the adult brain continues to produce new neurons (and other brain cells) and connections. The changes that occur in the adult brain are dependent on a person's behaviors as well as the environment in which they live, work, and enjoy their leisure time.[4] Age is also influential. In general, young brains tend to be more responsive to new experiences. However, older brains can also adapt as a result of learning, new experiences, and the formation of new memories.

How Can You Improve Your Neuroplasticity?

Learning environments that invite you to focus your attention and face new information and challenges can stimulate positive changes in the brain.[5] To stimulate your brain, you might try:

- Learning to play music.
- Learning a new language.
- Juggling.
- Challenging your brain with daily puzzles or tests.
- Learning to dance or mastering a TikTok choreography.
- Playing video games.

Neuroplasticity and Gaming

Many teens are delighted to discover that gaming can have positive effects on their brain development. One 2012 study showed that playing *Super Mario 64* significantly increases gray matter (which processes information) in the brain. However, not all games confer the same benefits. For instance, one 2018 study showed that first-person shooting games reduce gray matter in the hippocampus. This is because Super Mario players rely on the hippocampus for spatial memory, while those playing shooting games rely on non-spatial memory strategies.

Video Games Should Be Enjoyed in Moderation

Gaming may have benefits, but it is important to enjoy them moderately. Because computer games rewire the brain for instant gratification, they can become addictive very quickly. You may have noticed, for instance, that when you defeat an enemy in an action game, you get a rush of enjoyment. This rush is caused by a neurotransmitter called dopamine. When too much dopamine floods the brain, it inhibits your ability to feel pleasure, so you need to play more to fulfil your needs. Excess dopamine can also cause your frontal lobe to shrink, leading to moodiness, anxiety, and difficulties with school and work. Remember that during your teen years, your brain is still developing and that it is very susceptible to changes.[6]

CREATING A GROWTH MINDSET

In the introduction, we spoke about the importance of embracing a growth mindset. Now that you know that you can continue to learn and pick up new skills throughout your lifetime, it makes sense to embrace growth rather than remain in stagnation.

What Is the Difference Between Fixed and Growth Mindsets?

American Psychologist Carol Dweck, developed the concept of a growth mindset. She specializes in human motivation, aiming to understand why people succeed and what factors they can embrace if they wish to achieve their goals. Dweck postulates that there are two mindsets: a fixed and a growth mindset.

People who employ a fixed mindset believe that intelligence is static. This leads them to want to look smart and to:

- Avoid challenges.
- Evade obstacles.
- Devalue effort and hard work.

- Ignore useful negative feedback.
- Feel threatened by the success of other people.

Those with a growth mindset have a desire to learn and tend to:

- Embrace challenges and see them as an opportunity to improve.
- Persist even if things get difficult.
- See effort as the key to mastery.
- Learn from criticism.
- Find inspiration and aim to learn important lessons from the success of others.

It is probably easy to see how people with a growth mindset can achieve their full potential. It is impossible to become skilled at something if obstacles and hard work faze you. If you try to see challenges as something fun and exciting to overcome, there is so much you can achieve.

In her book, *Mindset: The New Psychology of Success*, Dweck explains why having a fixed mindset can be so tough.[7] When you believe that you are born with a specific amount of intelligence or a certain character, then you have to keep proving yourself. You evaluate every situation, asking yourself if you will look smart or stupid, if you will be accepted or rejected, if others will welcome or shun you. When you have a growth mindset, on the other hand you do not believe that you are simply "handed" a set of traits. "In this mindset, the hand you're dealt is just the starting point for development," says Dweck. There are so many qualities you can cultivate through effort.

Fixed Mindsets and Social Anxiety

Having a fixed mindset can make your social anxiety worse, since you may always be worrying about saying the right thing, having the right response, or looking the right way. Having a growth mindset can help you view mistakes as part of growing up and maturing. If you ask a parent or trusted adult about funny or embarrassing things that happened to them with friends in their teen years, you will probably notice how much fun they have recalling these times. By trying to protect yourself at all costs through perfectionism, you can miss out on making memories and learning the things that work (and those that are best avoided).

A Growth Mindset Can Help People Overcome Shyness

Psychologist Jennifer Beer, studied the way that growth of fixed mindsets can affect people with social anxiety by conducting a test on hundreds of people with this type of anxiety. She videoed pairs of people getting to know each other and asks observers to evaluate how they acted. Prior to the test, she measured participants' mindsets and levels of shyness.

The results showed that although shy people seemed anxious as a whole during the first few minutes of conversation, socially anxious people with a growth mindset came across as more pleasant to observers than socially anxious individuals with a fixed mindset. This is because although they were scared, they approached the situation as a challenge. Those with a fixed mindset saw the same event as a risk to be avoided.[8]

Kendis' Story

Kendis always felt he was born to dance. Some of the earliest videos featured him moving gracefully to dance music. By the time he was four, his mother, Sandra, had already enrolled him in pre-ballet. His teachers had wonderful things to say about his talent. Kendis seemed to have a natural flexibility and ability to learn new choreographies. He used to love performing for his family, and created many of his own choreographies for special occasions like Christmas and his parents' birthday.

When Kendis turned 11, however, things changed, and they did so dramatically. He started developing social anxiety and no longer wanted to perform for others—either at home or school. He also became very anxious about switching to pointe work (dancing "on his toes"). It felt painful and when he tried this technique, he would lose his balance. He felt that if he couldn't do pointe, and he didn't want to perform, perhaps it was because dancing was not for him.

Kendis didn't know it, but he was developing a fixed mindset that caused him to turn his back to dancing. It wasn't until his late teens, when he had already started college, that he was inspired to learn to dance again. He had struck up a friendship with a psychology professor, who first shared information about the growth mindset with him. Kendis signed up for night dance classes, started watching live ballet performances, and began dancing when he'd go out to clubs. He added modern dance to his repertoire, and made it a point to get on the dance floor, even if he was scared that others were watching him and feared they might think he didn't have any talent or that his moves were off.

As he moved from a fixed to a growth mindset, he began performing with a dance group, even though he would always feel a little jittery before the show started. He started with very small roles in the shows, but eventually accepted the opportunity to be a lead dancer when his teacher said he needed to let his talent shine. He would always feel on cloud nine afterwards, and he realized that his growth mindset had reunited him with his passion. Furthermore, he told himself that it really didn't matter if someone didn't like his moves. People don't have to like everything you do. All of us have artists, musicians, and actors we enjoy watching more than others. Opinions do not define you, and they definitely shouldn't separate you from the things that make you happy.

TAKING IT ONE STEP AT A TIME

Getting over social anxiety does not have to happen overnight. In Kendis' case, for instance, you may notice that he took various steps before feeling truly free of his fears. In Chapter Seven, we will go through exposure therapy, which involves facing your triggers little by little, until you start feeling more and more in control.

How Can Adopting a Growth Mindset Make Your Teen Years More Fun?

Having a growth mindset reduces the effect that perfectionism can have on your life. However, it can have many added bonuses that will help you fill more of the bottles we spoke about earlier. With a growth mindset you can:

- Discover a love of learning.
- Improve your grades at high school or college by trying new study techniques, creating a new study schedule, and starting to study for exams earlier.
- Try out adventurous things.
- Learn valuable lessons by taking feedback non-defensively.
- Use humor to reduce tension when you "don't get it right."

WHY IS FEEDBACK SO VALUABLE?

When you are older and work becomes one of your main responsibilities, you may find that your manager provides you with regular feedback. It can be hard to accept feedback with an open heart if you see it as an attack. The truth is that it is only human to enjoy hearing nice things about oneself. However, receiving honest opinions is priceless, since people often fear saying what is really on their mind to avoid hurting others or creating conflict.

When someone gives you feedback with a kind intention and respectful words, try to listen with an open heart. You can take time to reflect on what they said and consider making changes that can help you grow as a person, friend, student, and worker. Managers are taught to give employees feedback frequently because it is easier to correct a small mistake early, before it escalates or becomes a habit. Remember that you are separate from your actions or behaviors. They do not define you. Therefore, if there is a behavior you think you work on, this says nothing negative about your identity. Quite the contrary; it marks you as an open person who lets a growth mindset lead the way.

HOW CAN YOU DEVELOP A GROWTH MINDSET?

Below are seven steps you can take to develop a growth mindset.

1. **Ask yourself if you have a fixed or growth mindset.** There are many online quizzes that can help you see which mindset you may currently prefer. One easy test you can complete in minutes can be found on Big Life Journal.[9] A similar test can be found on WDHB.[10] If your results indicate you may have a fixed mindset, remember that you can move towards the growth mindset.

2. **Ask yourself which aspects of your life you feel a growth mindset would improve.** This will enable you to feel motivated to take steps to be more open to learning and change.

3. **Conduct some research on people who have learned to adopt a growth mindset.** Kobe Bryant, the American professional basketball player, who helped lead the Los Angeles Lakers win five championships, once said, "Everything negative—pressure, challenges—is all an opportunity for me to rise." Kobe faced many challenges along his stellar career. For instance, he ruptured his Achilles tendon in 2013 during a game but just four months later, he was already running and jumping, thanks to his hard work with the Lakers' head physical therapist, Judy Seto. Many questioned if he would ever return professionally, but just eight months after he was injured, he officially returned in a game against the Toronto Raptors.

4. **Change how you view failure.** Nothing is a better teacher than "getting it wrong." Thomas Edison once said, "I have not failed. I've just found 10,000 ways that won't work." His words show that he never let failure steer him off his course. Winston Churchill also hit the nail on

the head when he said, "Success is stumbling from failure to failure with no loss of enthusiasm." Your journal will be vital when it comes to this step. Whenever you feel that you have failed or made a mistake, write it down. Let a little time pass and go back to what you wrote, listing the things your mistake may have taught you.

5. **Be careful of labeling yourself or others, for good or bad, with "fixed mindset" terms.** For instance, saying someone is a "naturally talented" runner may be hurtful to someone else who is just starting out in this sport. These words reinforce a fixed mindset.

6. **Stop seeking approval from others.** Compliments are wonderful, but they should not be your main aim when performing tasks or reaching for goals. Whether someone thinks you're great or not, remember that it is an opinion. No matter how well you do something, someone may still think it's uncool. By contrast, you may do or create something you don't think is very good, and someone may love it. Either way, building a growth mindset is all about enjoying the process of learning, discovering things about yourself and others, learning new skills, honing abilities, and

committing to the work required to achieve success. Success does not have to be material. For instance, your goal could be to take part in a debate or to say yes the next time someone invites you out. Keep in mind that growth can be difficult, awkward, and even a little embarrassing. Allow yourself to feel these emotions, but try accepting the challenge anyway, keeping your mind on how good you will feel about yourself afterwards.

7. **Celebrate the growth of others.** It can be so liberating to feel true happiness when things go well for someone else. Be especially celebratory of people who achieve things they have found challenging at first. Use their success to inspire you to set the bar higher.

GROWTH MINDSET AFFIRMATIONS

Below are a few affirmations that can help you improve your mindset. Choose those you find useful and say them to yourself daily.

- "I have everything I need to make today a fantastic day."
- "I am living to my full potential."

- "I will let any challenges I encounter motivate me."
- "I trust my intuition."
- "I can let go of negative beliefs that have no evidence in fact."
- "I am excited about all the good things that can happen today."
- "I will learn something important today."
- "I am learning to value the journey."
- "I am strong enough to overcome challenges."
- "I will face challenges confidently."
- "I am confident and good things come my way."
- "Today, I will embrace positive thoughts and language."
- "I will do something good for someone else today."
- "I will encourage others to strive for their goals."
- "I am letting go of others' judgments."
- "I liberate myself with forgiveness."
- "I accept my flaws because all human beings have them."
- "I will celebrate the success of others today."

CREATING A GROWTH MINDSET VISION BOARD

If you love working with visuals, you may enjoy creating a growth mindset vision board that can serve as inspiration. To do so, start with a basic layout that indicates the main ideas you want your board to contain. Plan how you will divide your board up and make sure your poster or cardboard background is large enough to contain all your ideas. Next, get creative, using a blend of visuals, quotes, graphics, and other elements. You can print your quotes and images on colored paper, create your own drawings, or use photographs you can print or cut out from magazines. Update your vision board regularly.

In this chapter, we highlighted the plastic nature of the brain. People are not born with a fixed amount of knowledge. They can continue to grow and learn, even in their senior years. The fact that the brain is malleable is a great reason to adopt a growth mindset.

Believing that you are born with fixed talents and skills can be damaging. It can put you off your goals and dreams and stagnate you. To cultivate a growth mindset, don't seek others' approval and make an effort to find value from every mistake, every small "failure." Celebrate the growth of others and remember to exercise self-kindness and to utilize humor; it's a great weapon against awkwardness and a good laugh can be so liberating. Concentrate on the journey, using self-affirmations and mood boards to keep you focused.

Now that you know the importance of change and flexibility, it's time to focus on managing your emotions. In Chapter Five, we will share essential coping strategies that will help you deal with overwhelming or powerful emotions.

I AM PAYING IT FORWARD

"We're all in this together. Each and every one of us can make a difference by giving back."

— *BEYONCÉ*

One of the central strategies involved in DBT is 'coping ahead' to help you reduce difficult emotions and relieve your anxiety.

Imagine you're going to a party. It's going to be noisy and crowded, and you know it will trigger your social anxiety. To cope with this in advance, you can start by describing the situation you're worried about and naming the emotions that come up for you. From there, you can decide on the coping strategies you could use to help you on the day – for example, maybe you'll go outside every time you feel yourself getting over-whelmed.

Coping ahead can be used for all kinds of situations – perhaps you want to check the route to a particular place in advance, or make a backup plan in case you miss your bus; perhaps you want to read reviews before you sign up to something to make sure you know exactly what you're getting into.

Reviews are a really useful tool when it comes to reducing your anxiety about something – seeing what other people thought of it before you commit will help you visualize what's troubling you and come up with strategies to deal with it.

Reviews are also how you'll find the resources you need to help you with your anxiety. And this is your opportunity to help other young people like you...

By leaving a review of this book on Amazon, you can help other people who are struggling with anxiety to find the tools that will help them cope.

Your review will act as a signpost showing other teenagers that people like them have used the strategies in this book to help them – and that will pave the way for them to access those strategies for themselves. Essentially, you'll be helping other people like you to cope ahead by pointing them in the direction of the tools they need to do so.

Thank you for taking the time to help me with this – I know we can help more people overcome their anxiety this way, and I'm thrilled that you want to be part of that mission.

Scan the QR code below to leave your review:

5

I CAN MANAGE MY EMOTIONS

> "*This might surprise you, but one of the best ways to manage your emotions is simply to experience that emotion and let it run its course.*"
>
> — KIM L. GRATZ

When you have social anxiety, you can experience an array of emotions when you are with others, including fear. You may dread being rejected, or saying or doing something embarrassing. You might also feel overwhelmed when you are in the presence of authority figures, or feel uncomfortable when someone asks you questions. Sometimes, it can seem like everyone around you is hostile or quick to judge. Once the occasion is over and you are alone, you can feel ashamed about being "different" from others and engage in intense self-criticism, second-guessing yourself and obsessing about what you could have done differently. This can lead to emotional overwhelm.

SIGNS YOU MAY BE EMOTIONALLY OVERWHELMED

If your emotions are getting the better of you, you may have one or more of the following symptoms:[1]

- Difficulties with remembering, reasoning, and solving problems.
- Being more irritable.
- Feeling "on the edge."
- An increased heart rate or chest pain.
- More frequent headaches.
- Teeth grinding and/or jaw clenching.
- Feeling fatigued.
- Feeling more anxious, or depressed.
- Having gastrointestinal issues.
- Sleeping more or less than usual.
- Having changes in your eating habits.
- Feeling dizzy.
- Shortness of breath.

COMMON TRIGGERS FOR EMOTIONAL OVERLOAD

If you have social anxiety, some situations can be particularly triggering when it comes to your emotions. These can include:

- Having to speak or perform in public.
- Receiving unwanted physical contact or attention.
- Being in the presence of emotionally intense people or groups.
- Taking on too many responsibilities at once.
- Moving to a new school or making another major transition that involves distancing yourself from your current sources of support.

SOCIAL ANXIETY AND EMOTIONAL REGULATION

In Chapter Two, we broached the subject of cognitive distortions and how they can make things seem much worse than they are. People with social anxiety sometimes have to battle two additional challenges: "emotional hyperreactivity" and difficulties with emotional regulation.

What Is Emotional Hyperreactivity?

People with emotional hyperreactivity can have strong thoughts, feelings, and reactions that are more intense than those the average person might have. They may also:[2]

- Experience positive emotions (like happiness) more intensely.
- Feel the pain of being criticized, rejected, teased, or judged much more powerfully than most people around them.
- Fail to notice their mood shifts and get "blindsided" by their own emotions.
- Have powerful emotions that seem to come out of nowhere.
- Have blow-ups when they feel emotionally overwhelmed.
- Find it hard to rid their mind of a specific thought or idea.
- Find it difficult to relax, even when they are on vacation.
- Have low self-esteem because of their emotional reactivity.
- Encounter sleep difficulties because they can't stop thoughts and worries from running through their head.

In essence, if you have SAD, you may appraise social situations in a way that transforms "harmless" social cues into personal threats. This can lead you to see others as critical and to feel like you are unable to function well in a social setting.

Social Anxiety and Emotional Regulation

Effective emotional regulation enables you to reduce your emotional reactions to situations that are stressful and anxiety-inducing. If you have SAD, you may find it harder to exercise this skill because you may perceive the words and actions of others as menacing.

EMOTIONAL REACTIVITY AND THE BRAIN

In Chapter One, we mentioned that people with SAD can have a more active amygdala. Typically, for instance, teens and adults who look at images of "harsh faces" have a powerful response in the amygdala and a greater likelihood of developing negative thoughts. The stronger the symptoms of this disorder are, the stronger your reaction can be. In one study published in the journal *Archives of General Psychiatry*, researchers found that people with SAD can:[3]

1. Experience elevated negative emotions to social threats.
2. Show differences in the parts of the brain involved in cognitive control (the mind's ability to inhibit automatic responses and respond flexibly so that their goals can be achieved).

When it comes to attention to social threats, people with SAD can follow a pattern of "vigilance and control." This means they can be extra-sensitive to potential threats. Once they feel threatened, they can turn their attention away from the cause of their fears, avoiding others as a way of protecting themselves. In the long run, avoidance can result in the reduction of your social circle and greater isolation. The results of the study do not mean that people with SAD cannot regulate their emotions. They simply show that they may find it challenging to do so.

How Can People With SAD Regulate Their Emotions?

In a 2020 study published in the journal *Biological Psychiatry: Cognitive Neuroscience and Neuroimaging*, researchers found that two emotional regulation strategies can be useful for people with SAD:[4]

- **Reappraisal:** This strategy involves reframing an event to reduce the negative emotions you feel and talking to yourself, so you can feel better about yourself or a situation.[5] For instance, if your buddy can't make it to your house as planned, you can reframe your disappointment by telling yourself things like, "It's a pity JJ couldn't come over, but I can use this time to start working on that big essay that's due in a few days." We spoke a little about reframing negative thoughts into positive ones in Chapter Two.

To benefit from this strategy, you can ask yourself useful questions like:

1. Are there any positive outcomes that can result from this situation?
2. Am I grateful for any part of this situation?
3. What did I learn from this situation?
4. How did I grow from this situation?

- **Acceptance:** This strategy is a component of mindfulness practice. Instead of trying to reframe a situation (as occurs during reappraisal), acceptance involves actively and fully experiencing thoughts, emotions, and sensations openly and non-judgmentally as they change from moment to moment. You don't need to make any attempt to change or avoid them.

Both reappraisal and acceptance involve attention control. There is a big difference between them, however. Reappraisal involves taking a new perspective to reinterpret a situation, while acceptance involves disengaging from typical patterns of reactivity and other negative thought processes.

The researchers concluded that for people with social anxiety, reappraisal might require more effort and resources than acceptance. This is because it involves taking on another perspective, selecting an appropriate way to reframe the situation, and other skills (which can be particularly challenging for people with severe symptoms of SAD). Acceptance and mindfulness, on the other hand, do not require as much effort. As always, it is advisable to try both strategies, and see which works best for you.

An Example of Acceptance and Mindfulness at Work

In Chapter Two, we also described how mindfulness work. Below is an example of how you can actively employ this strategy when you are feeling social anxiety:

You are invited to a party and decide to accept to give yourself a little "push." When you arrive, your friend introduces you to everyone, and you have a seat. You see someone looking at you and wonder if they find what you are wearing strange. Someone asks you if you do sports, and you tell them you play football, but are worried they will ask you more questions. You are worried you might do something like spit when you're talking, blush, or struggle to find the right words to say. You feel like telling your friend that you want to leave.

Instead of giving in to your instinct to avoid your thoughts and emotions, you take a mindful, accepting approach. You pay attention to the way your body is responding to what it perceives as a threat. You notice that your heart is going faster and that you are breathing through your mouth.

While the others are engaged in lively conversation, you do some belly breathing and focus on the air pushing your belly forward and back. You are aware of your discomfort, but you don't push it away. Instead of telling yourself you are "silly" or that your fears are "unfounded," you simply allow your thoughts and emotions to exist.

You tell yourself that these thoughts and emotions are like a wave. Right now you are at the peak of the wave but in a while, you will float over it and come out safe on the other side. You tell yourself that there is nothing wrong with your emotions and that they do not define you. You remind yourself that it is okay to feel scared, awkward, or ashamed.

You begin to feel a bit more in control. Thanks to controlled breathing, your heart rate has come down, and you are breathing through your nose. You are ready to feel positive emotions, but you won't repress the negative ones or hide them. You allow yourself to be silent for a while. After a while, you find someone that is interesting to talk to. Someone else joins your conversation. You aim to enjoy the interchange of ideas, giving yourself fully to the moment and the people you are engaging with. When you say something you think is silly, you use humor to make light of it, or simply rephrase what you wanted to say. Because you accept yourself, you are less aware of how others perceive you. You remember this conversation a few days later, and are motivated to see your new friends again.

GROUNDING TECHNIQUES

When you are experiencing anxiety and other uncomfortable techniques, you can try a few grounding exercises to bring you back to the present moment. Below are a few that you may find helpful:

I The 5-4-3-2-1 Technique

This technique uses the five senses, so you can concentrate on the present and avoid the barrage of anxious thoughts that can stand in the way of progress. Before starting, take a few deep breaths until you achieve a calmer slight. Then, proceed to the following steps:[6]

5. See: Acknowledge five things you see around you. Try noticing small, detailed things like the shadow cast by a lamp, the colors in a painting on the wall, or the way a pet's belly rises and falls as they are sleeping.

4. Touch: Acknowledge four things you can touch in your surroundings. You can simply notice the way the material of your shirt feels on your body, touch your hair, take a notebook and feel its sparkly surface, or gently touch the keys on your keyboard.

3. Hear: Acknowledge three things you can hear. These can include your dog snoring, music playing, and the sound of your air conditioner.

2. Smell: Acknowledge two things around you with a fragrance or aroma. You might pick up a candle, or open a jar of cookies and breathe its appealing scent in.

1. Acknowledge one thing near you that you can taste. It might be cinnamon-flavored dental floss, a cup of tea, or the cookie in that jar!

II Body Awareness

This technique aims to increase your awareness of your bodily sensations. Before starting, practice belly breathing for a few minutes, until you enter a more relaxed state. Next, follow these steps:

1. Place both your feet on the ground, wiggling your toes and arching and curling your foot. Take note of all the sensations that arise in your feet. Stomp on the ground and jump, once again noticing how your feet feel.
2. Next, it's time to work on your hands. Close your hands into fists, then release them, ensuring no tension is left in your fingers. Repeat this various times.
3. Press your palms against each other, noticing the resistance in your hands and arms.
4. Rub your palms together quickly, noticing the warmth that arises.
5. Lift your hands to the sky, enjoying a wonderful stretch. Sustain this pose for about

five seconds, then bring your hands to the sides
of your hips and relax.

6. Take a few deep breaths and notice the sense of
calm that has returned to your body.

III Mental Exercises

These exercises keep your mind busy so that uncomfortable thoughts and emotions don't take over. You
can try:

1. Counting backwards from 100 by six.
2. Naming all your family members, their
   birthdays, and their favorite hobby.
3. Reading a line of text backwards.
4. Drawing an object in the air or on glass using
   your finger. It could be something simple like a
   leaf or something more complex, like your
   bedroom, with all its furniture and decorative
   items.

IV Categories

Choose a few of the categories below and name as many items as you can that belong to them:

- Cakes
- Famous influencers
- Talented TikTokers
- Series
- Books
- Bands
- Football teams
- Fashion designers
- Artists
- Authors

V Journaling and Social Anxiety

We have suggested keeping a journal several times in this book, since it can be especially useful for strategies such as reframing negative core beliefs and cognitive distortions. Recent studies show that journaling has various benefits for people with social anxiety:

- **It sharpens your critical thinking skills.**
Research published in the *International Journal of Higher Education* shows that journal writing helps students develop their critical thinking skills.[7] In the study, this activity helped participants reason, think logically, and evaluate different options to come to a decision. All these skills can come in handy when you are trying to reappraise a negative situation.
- **It helps you identify patterns of behavior you can work on.**[8] For instance, you may notice that when somebody teases you, you leave the group you are with. In time, this can point out that you are missing out on good times. You can reappraise the situation and try to see "banter" as a normal part of getting close to someone, or find a way to assertively set your limits if you feel that someone is crossing them. You may decide to simply observe the pattern and wait until you are strong enough to do something about it.
- **It helps prevent and reduces anxiety.** A 2018 study showed that journaling can mitigate mental distress, increase wellbeing, and enhance your physical health.[9]

How to Use a Journal to Soothe Social Anxiety

If possible, get into the habit of using your journal every evening or as often as you can. Around five to 15 minutes is great to start off with, though some people enjoy journaling for longer. Find a peaceful, quiet spot in your home. Put on some soothing music if you like and use an essential oil diffuser with a scent like lavender to put you in a calm mood.[10] Once you're ready, follow these steps:[11]

1. **Write down the situations that are causing you worry.** For instance, you might write:

- "I am worried I will start blushing or sweating when someone starts asking me questions at the party."
- "My mind might go completely blank when the teacher asks me to give my speech."
- "I am worried that my sister's friends will criticize me when they come over."

2. **Next, explore the degree to which your own thoughts and beliefs may be shaping your worries.** Ask yourself questions like:

- "How likely is it that the others will notice my hands are sweating when we are discussing our group project?"
- "What is the very worst thing that could happen, and would it matter in a few years' time?"
- "Is there any way I can look at my fears differently, so I can lessen their power over my life?"

Dealing with a tough situation: In the situation in which you have to present your English project before class , the very worst thing that could happen could be that you get so nervous you forget what you had planned to say.

In this case, come up with a plan of attack! For instance, you might say to your teacher, "I'm sorry, I've gone blank. I'm a bit nervous. Could someone else go before me, so I can calm down?"

Remember that when you don't "perform" the way you want to, making a joke about it or simply letting others know you are nervous can calm the entire situation. If you smile and tell your classmates, "Argh! I hate it when this happens, but I'm feeling a bit anxious. I need a little time," you might be surprised at how empathetic they actually are. You might also be pleased to learn that it's hard for many of them to speak in public or talk to new people. They may simply be good at hiding their fears.

Anyone that judges you for this moment may be masking their own fears or insecurities. Most people know how stressful public speaking can be, and more than one person will be grateful if someone else points this out in class. Even if you feel so flustered you are unable to give your speech at all that day, this probably won't affect your final grade, your chance of getting into college, or your life as a whole. It's just one scary moment, and you're allowed to have those, as we all are.

Understanding that the worst-case scenario actually isn't life-shattering can instantly render a "monster" problem powerless, especially when you start feeling more in control of your reactions. Don't be afraid to share your "weaknesses" with others, because doing so can be a strength. It enables others to relate to you and shows you are a human being with your own fears, insecurities, and worries.

3. Try to see each concern differently, writing down positive possible outcomes and finding meaning from each experience.
4. Write down your strengths, and then see if they can help you in these situations. For instance, you may be empathetic to others. How

about directing empathy towards yourself, so that you see that nerves are human and that it is okay to take your time, ask for a break, or ask for help.

5. Decide how you will prepare to tackle these situations. For instance, you might decide to summarize your talk into main points and write these down on small cards. You may speak to trusted members of your class first and let them know you are worried, so you feel more comfortable about asking your teacher for a break if you need to. You may also embrace stress management techniques in the days leading up to your talk, and engage in mindfulness meditation on the morning of your speech. During the class, you may engage in controlled breathing or mindfulness exercise to keep your mind in the present moment.

When you have social anxiety, managing your emotions can seem like an insurmountable obstacle. In this chapter, we revealed that emotional regulation is possible for people with social anxiety. We also showed that there is more than one way to control emotional overwhelm. You can try reframing negative thoughts and beliefs into more positive ones, though you may find mindful acceptance more useful.

Journaling is another powerful means of understanding yourself more and of seeing your triggers with a greater perspective. In Chapter Six, we will dive right into another exciting challenge: questioning oneself! Once again, your journal will be a powerful tool when it comes to identifying and challenging irrational thoughts and understanding more about the situations that can stress you out.

6

I CAN QUESTION MYSELF

> "*Ask yourself the hard questions, never stop asking, and allow your answers to change as you do.*"
>
> — COLIN WRIGHT

P eople with social anxiety often know that their anxiety is irrational and is not based on fact. However, it can be very hard to battle the barrage of emotions and thoughts that can flood your brain when you are contemplating social interaction. You already know a few reasons why these anxious thoughts arise— including hyperactivity of the amygdala. You also know that reappraisal and acceptance can help you escape negative thought patterns because the brain is plastic, and you can learn and practice the skills you need to keep these patterns in check.

WHY IS QUESTIONING YOURSELF IMPORTANT?

Many successful people stress the importance of questioning themselves. They are wise enough to know that when you are a leader or manager, people may sometimes be afraid to question you or give honest feedback. This is why top managers find ways to receive feedback confidentially (for instance, through anonymous feedback forms). They also make it a point to take frequent pauses, so they can question what they are getting right or wrong. Strong leaders trust their intuition, and they listen to their gut feeling, even when it is telling them something negative.

Strong thoughts often feel like facts, but they are not. By frequently challenging your assumptions and asking yourself questions, you can consider things from a more objective perspective.

A LIFE LESSON FROM VINCENT VAN GOGH

Vincent Van Gogh, the post-impressionist painter who is famed for paintings like *The Starry Night* and *Vase with Fifteen Sunflowers*, was plagued with self-doubt.[1] However, he chose to battle the negative thoughts that raced through his head through creativity. He once said, "If you hear a voice within you say you cannot paint, then by all means paint and that voice will be silenced." His words are a reminder that you can't really move forward if you try to avoid the things you fear by hiding, isolating yourself, or freezing on the spot. When you find that you are telling yourself you cannot do something, you have two ways to respond. The first is to fall prey to negative thoughts and believe they are right. The second is to have a strong desire to prove these thoughts wrong. Which choice do you think will be most beneficial to you?

HOW ARE ANXIETY AND IRRATIONAL THINKING RELATED?

Some types of irrational thoughts that are logically irrational can lead to difficulties with coping and can cause anxiety symptoms to arise. Irrational thoughts can take the following forms:[2]

- **Unwanted images, thoughts, or memories.**
  You may see yourself behaving in a specific way in a social setting—for instance, you might see yourself blurting out information everyone

laughs at. You may also vividly imagine people looking at you with disapproval or disgust.

- **Strange worries.** You may suddenly find yourself worrying about something without an obvious trigger for it. For instance, you might suddenly feel everyone thinks you're boring, or develop a feeling that things are not okay with friends or other social groups. These worries may pop up randomly or be recurrent.
- **A fear that you are losing control.**

The following are typical irrational thoughts someone with social anxiety may have:[3]

- "If I go out, I'll do or say something dumb, and I won't ever be invited to another party again."
- "I don't know enough people at this party. I'm leaving!"
- "I can't join a conversation, as others may think I am butting in."
- "They will notice I am breathing funny."
- "I just want to crawl into a hole to avoid everyone here."
- "I look strange and everyone will think I'm odd."
- "I want to stay home for days, so I don't have to see anyone."

- "How on earth do people manage at parties?"
- "I hope I don't run into people from school at the mall."
- (At the mall): "Oh no. There are my classmates. I hope they can't see me!"

HOW CAN YOU CHALLENGE IRRATIONAL THOUGHTS? A PRACTICAL EXERCISE

You can start challenging irrational thoughts by asking yourself the following questions and by using your journal to answer and analyze them:[4]

1. Have previous experiences shown me that this fear is not completely true?
2. When I am feeling differently, how might I perceive this situation?
3. Is there any evidence that what I am thinking is not actually occurring?
4. Have I ever jumped to conclusions in the past, then realized things were not the way I had initially assumed?
5. How would a friend or family member perceive this situation?
6. What are some other ways I can think about this situation?

7. Even if there is some truth to my thoughts, is it helpful for me to think like this?

You can then summarize your new perspective. For instance, for the thought, "They're all going to laugh at me at the party," you might write: At the last party I went to, I felt really shy at first, but my friend John introduced me to a couple of his friends, and they were really nice. I spoke a little about music with his friend, Stewart, and I find out Stewart played in a band. Stewart told me he would be playing at his friend, Tim's party, and that I should go."

Things to Keep in Mind When Challenging Irrational Thoughts

Most people aren't taught to challenge their thoughts, and it can be very difficult to do at first. Below are a few considerations to keep in mind when you start:

- You don't have to challenge every single negative thought.
- In order to build your confidence, start with thoughts that aren't too upsetting. It can also help to choose a moment in which you feel neutral, not one in which your anxiety is high.

- Use your journal to capture your thoughts on paper instead of running over the same thoughts over and over again.
- Try challenging your thoughts with a trusted friend or family member. They might have interesting perspectives that can help you view situations more objectively.
- Challenge one thought at a time instead of taking on too many at once.
- Plan to do something relaxing after questioning your thoughts so that new perspectives have time to settle.

Challenging your thoughts may be less efficient than taking a mindfulness approach and accepting them as they are, eventually moving on from them. Everyone is an individual and throughout your journey with social anxiety, it pays to use the strategies that work. This doesn't mean you should give up the first time. Have a few tries at challenging your thoughts and see how helpful the process is for you.

SHARPENING CONFLICT RESOLUTION SKILLS

If you have social anxiety, then one of the things that may most worry you, is how to handle yourself in conflicts with others. Conflicts can be very stressful because they call upon you to be your strongest self; to assert your limits, listen actively to what others have to say, and work collaboratively towards a solution.

Conflicts can be beneficial in many ways. For instance, they can inspire you and others to produce new ideas, build empathy and understanding, and boost creativity.[5] In order to build and strengthen your relationship with others, analyze your conflict management style and question if you could benefit from using additional styles in specific situations.

What Is Your Conflict Management Style?

There is no single ideal conflict management style. In fact, you may use one or more when you are dealing with conflict. Understanding the main styles you prefer and being aware of the other ones, however, can help you resolve conflicts more efficiently when they arise.[6] Doing so can make you feel more comfortable when you are called upon to work collaboratively with classmates or get along with others in a group. If you employ handy conflict resolution skills and keep things respectful and solution-based, you can avoid simply running away from conflict or isolating yourself to evade it.

The Five Main Conflict Management Styles

Most people use one or more of the following conflict management styles:

Collaborative Style

People with a collaborative style approach conflict as a way to ensure that everyone is happy with the outcome. Conflicts are viewed as a team, with all players working together to achieve a goal. This minimizes negative feelings and enables all sides to feel like they are being heard. When you take part in discussions with a person with a collaborative style, it is easier to feel less defensive and more focused on solving the problem at hand, while maintaining respect and valuing others' feelings.

Competing Style

People who compete with others simply want to "win" a conflict instead of finding a "win-win" solution. This style can be useful in a limited range of circumstances (for instance, when you're participating in a school debate, and you need to win this round to make it to the finals). However, when you are in a conflict with friends or family, this style can put people on the defense and make them feel that their feelings, needs, and desires don't matter.

People sometimes employ this style as a way to defend themselves. The downside is that although they may win (or achieve the outcome they want), others may see them as selfish, unreasonable, or unpleasant to deal with. Others may accede simply to avoid fighting, not because they are happy with the final outcome.

Avoidant Style

People who favor this style tend to be unassertive and uncooperative, withdrawing from conflict and often seeking distance. This style can be useful in a high-tension situation; one in which everyone can benefit from time to cool down. However, if every time you have a conflict with someone you withdraw emotionally or physically, it can lead to long-term avoidance of issues that need to be resolved if a relationship or friendship is to move forward.

Accommodating Style

This style involves sacrificing your needs or wants (to some extent) in order to satisfy others. It can be useful once in a while, especially when the outcome is not so important or when the other person frequently accommodates your needs. However, if you accede to others' demands or prioritize their needs too often, you can later feel angry, resentful, or even ashamed that you have not "stood up for yourself." This can lead to passive-aggressive behavior, in which you express your negative feelings indirectly instead of openly addressing them.

Compromising Style

This style involves finding a mutually acceptable solution that partially satisfies all parties to the conflict while still maintaining assertiveness and cooperation. This style works well to solve a small issue quickly. Its downside is that the matter may be "settled" without the parties being truly satisfied with the result.

SOCIAL ANXIETY AND AVOIDANCE

Research published in the journal *Behavior Therapy* showed that higher levels of social anxiety are linked to interpersonal styles reflecting less assertiveness, more avoidance of conflicts and of expressing emotion, and greater interpersonal dependency.[7] However, as is the case with other behavioral skills, learning to negotiate conflicts effectively can be learned.

What Does Successful Conflict Resolution Depend on?

Dealing with conflicts in a healthy, productive manner involves:[8]

- **Managing stress while remaining calm.** When a conflict arises, it is important to maintain a respectful tone and use open (rather than closed) body language. For instance, you should avoid crossing your arms against your chest, clenching your fists, or spreading your body for stability. To de-escalate conflicts, show your palms, try to relax your body, make sure your eye contact is just right (not overly intense), and use physical touch if appropriate.
- **Controlling your emotions.** If necessary, try a little breathing or take a little break if you find you are overwhelmed by your emotions. Regularly practicing mindfulness will sharpen your emotional awareness and enable you to stop feelings like fear or anger from escalating.
- **Listening actively to others.** This involves listening to their words, observing their body language, and showing you are really hearing them and their concerns.
- **Being aware of and accepting of differences.** Everyone has their own conflict style, as well as

their values, thoughts, and opinions. Make sure the person you are discussing an issue with feels respected and valued. Recognize and respond to matters that are very important to them.

In any conflict, qualities like the ability to compromise, avoid punishing or withdrawing your love from others, and being ready to forgive and forget, are helpful. Humor can also play a critical role in reducing tension and reminding the other person that you care for each other and that you should fix the problem and move on, so you can create many more great memories.

When engaged in conflict, focus on the present instead of bringing up past hurts. Avoid language such as "You always," or "You never," which can make the other person feel defensive. Finally, avoid behavior that "punishes" a friend or loved one. Withdrawing your friendship from them and refusing to talk to them could cause them great pain. It is fine to take a little break if an argument gets too heated, but closing the door behind you can slowly erode at a friendship or relationship.

Sam's Story

Sam had been best friends with his schoolmate, Joey, since they were three years old. Now that they were in high school, they enjoyed each other's company greatly, and could often communicate without words. Just a look or glance from Joey could make Sam burst into laughter, and vice versa. Sam loved Joey because he was trustworthy and knew how to keep a secret. He would also give him practical advice without getting too "sappy."

However, every time they would argue or on occasions when Sam wanted to respectfully talk about something Joey had done that hurt him, Joey would refuse to discuss the issue and leave the room, often banging the door behind him. Sam would try to contact him later in the day by text, but Joey wouldn't answer. He would then refuse to talk to him at school, sometimes for an entire week—despite the fact that they hadn't argued over anything deep and intense. Joey avoided conflicts (and talking about them) at all costs. Then, when he was "over it," he would suddenly send Sam a funny text or message and the friendship would resume as if nothing had happened. When Sam broached the subject they had been arguing about, Joey would just summarize why he thought he was right and quickly change the subject.

This went on for a few years, but one day, Sam stopped trying; his energy had been completely depleted and he felt like he was constantly compromising his needs to keep the friendship going. He would still talk to Joey when he saw him at school or at parties. However, Sam avoided telling Joey how he felt or letting him know when he didn't like something Joey had done, because he knew it would only lead to avoidant behavior, awkwardness, and pain.

Joey didn't know it, but Sam was slowly tiring of their relationship. When his mom asked him why he didn't hang around Joey as much as before, he answered, "I feel our friendship isn't equal. It feels like I always have to walk on eggshells so he doesn't get angry, and I don't like that he doesn't answer my texts or calls when a day or two has passed."

Over time, Sam began getting closer to his other class-mates and began seeing Joey as more of an acquaintance. He still liked him and when they were together, the chemistry and laughs still flowed. However, he realized he could not keep hurting himself by expecting Sam to change. He also realized that Sam's avoidant behavior was something that caused him too much hurt and discomfort to withstand constantly. There is a saying that his grandmother used to tell him that rang true. "You've got to get up and leave the table when love's no longer being served."

FAQ: What Does Being Assertive Mean?

Being assertive is different from being passive, aggressive, or passive-aggressive.[9] The difference between these communication styles is as follows:

- Assertive communication involves expressing your point of view in a clear, direct manner, while respecting others.
- Passive communication often involves acceding to everyone else's demands, putting one's own wants and needs on the back burner. Some people who use this communication style speak quietly, use passive phrases such as "only if you don't mind," and try excessively to "keep the peace."
- Aggressive communication involves forcing opinions on others, maximizing one's needs (and minimize the needs of others), refusing to compromise, and damaging others' self-esteem.
- People with a passive-aggressive style can agree to others' demands, saying one thing and behaving in another manner. Passive-aggressive behavior includes resisting cooperation, procrastination, intentionally committing errors, or being sarcastic to others. This behavior occurs because one is secretly angry about having sacrificed one's needs for others.

STRATEGIES FOR BEING ASSERTIVE

To be more assertive, try to find "the right balance" between asserting your needs and acknowledging those of others. You can achieve this by:

- Using clear language to say what you want or need.
- Telling the other person how you feel in an honest and direct way, and listening to their thoughts and ideas as well.
- Using open body language (looking the person in the eye, relaxing your face, and nodding once in a while to show you are hearing them).
- Using "I" instead of "you" statements as much as possible to reduce defensiveness.
- Practicing often, as assertiveness is a skill you can refine over time.

PAYING IT FORWARD

Another way to challenge yourself is to aim to do one good deed every day (or on a regular basis). A study by researchers at the University of British Columbia has shown that keeping busy with acts of kindness can help people who have social anxiety mingle with others more easily.[10] Giving to others is known to boost happiness and can lead to a positive perception of other people and the world at large.

In a study, 115 undergraduate college students were randomly assigned to one of three groups for a month. The first group performed acts of kindness (such as doing a classmate's dishes, donating to a good cause, or mowing a neighbor's lawn). The second group only took part in social interactions, without performing altruistic deeds. The third group participated in no specific activities; all they had to do was record their activities every day. The results showed that the group that actively lent others a helping hand had a greater overall reduction in their desire to avoid social situations. Giving helped them counter the fear of rejection, and reduced their anxiety and distress.

Embracing challenges is an important part of moving forward. It helps you avoid stagnation, pulls you out of your comfort zone, and enables you to pick up life skills that will help you now and in your adulthood. In this chapter, we presented four main challenges: reframing irrational thoughts into rational ones, honing your conflict resolution skills, learning to express yourself assertively, and performing acts of service for others. While you don't have to brave all these challenges at once, trying at least one before you go to the next chapter will make you feel that you are making positive strides in your journey to better social relationships.

7

I CAN PUSH MYSELF

> " *"Avoidance is the best short-term strategy to escape conflict, and the best long-term strategy to ensuring suffering."*

— BRENDON BURCHARD

Exposure therapy is a "gold standard" treatment for most types of phobias, as well as for social anxiety. The basic idea behind it is that you cannot control your fears if you keep running away from them. However, facing your fears "all at once" can be overwhelming so instead, people are encouraged to do so little by little.

Phobias provide a good example of how exposure therapy works. Imagine you were afraid of dogs because as a child, you experienced a difficult or traumatic experience with one. Exposure therapy would involve gradually and repeatedly exposing you to dogs until your body broke the association between them and the emotion of fear. Typically, you would start by listing down a series of situations in which you might encounter dogs, and rating these experiences from most to least intense. For instance, you might find being with a puppy lower-intensity than being with an adult dog. You might prefer to be with a calm dog in your friend's home, than to interact with dogs in a public space. Your therapist would then expose you to the lowest-rated situation on your list and help you adapt to the uncomfortable sensations and emotions you might encounter. Little by little, you could work your way up the list. For some people, exposure therapy can give them successful results in a matter of hours. For others, the therapy may take several sessions.

EXPOSURE THERAPY AND SOCIAL ANXIETY

For most people, there is no way around working on group projects, attending important family events, and/or meeting new people. However, embracing all these situations at once can leave you in a state of panic if you have a high level of social anxiety. As is the case with someone who has a specific phobia, doing the thing you fear the most (for instance, giving a speech in public) may not be the best way to gradually dissociate your fear from social situations.

How Does Exposure Therapy for Social Anxiety Work?

Exposure therapy usually involves five essential steps.[1]

Step One: As is the case with phobias, harnessing the benefits of exposure therapy begins by listing the social situations that can cause you anxiety. You can use a zero-to-ten-point system (with zero being used for the lowest-anxiety situations and 10 for the highest), or you can use words ratings (no anxiety, low anxiety, moderate anxiety, high anxiety, very high anxiety). Once you have listed all the situations that may cause you distress, put them in order (from high to low or vice versa). Your list might look something like this:[2]

- Going to a party where I will encounter people I don't know well. Rating: Very high.
- Addressing my class when my teacher asks me to present my work. Rating: Very high.
- Having a job interview. Rating: Very High.
- Performing onstage. Rating: Very High.
- Going on a date. Rating: Very High.

- Eating out with people I don't know well. Rating: Very high.
- Entering a room where people are already seated. Rating: High.
- Starting a conversation. Rating: High.
- Inviting people to do something. Rating: High.
- Taking part in a work meeting or discussing a group project with classmates. Rating: High.
- Being assertive. Rating: High.
- Having coffee with my classmates. Rating: Moderate.
- Ordering food. Rating: Moderate.
- Making eye contact while talking. Rating: Moderate.
- Writing in front of others (for instance, filling in a form). Rating: Moderate.
- Returning purchases to a store. Rating: Low.
- Using a public bathroom. Rating: Low.
- Having coffee with my close friends. Rating: Low.
- Going to school. Rating: Low.
- Talking on the phone. Rating: Low.

Step Two: Choose a low-anxiety task and try it out. For instance, you might challenge yourself to call a classmate and ask a question about your homework, or simply talk about common interests. If when you set about to perform this task, you find that it is too hard, choose another low-rated activity instead.

Step Three: Do the activity or remain in the social situation until your anxiety is reduced.

Step Four: Repeat the activity various times until it becomes easy. Watch your list become shorter!

Step Five: Reflect on your experience and think of what you learned. You may notice, for instance, that some of your worst fears did not occur.

Tip One: People with social anxiety can sometimes use "safety behaviors." For instance, if you feel embarrassed when you start conversations, you may fiddle with your mobile while you are talking to avoid eye contact or to calm yourself down. Try to give yourself fully to the activity. Relying on safety behaviors can reduce the efficiency of exposure therapy. If you brave the challenges of exposure therapy head-on, your confidence will grow as you brave smaller (then larger) challenges throughout your journey.

TYPICAL SAFETY BEHAVIORS TO AVOID

Be aware of safety behaviors you might use to avoid the full effects of exposure therapy.[3] These include:

- Going to a party but sitting in the back of the room.
- Taking on a role that enables you to avoid social interaction (for instance, at a dinner party, you might head for the kitchen and make drinks for everyone, so you don't have to interact with them).
- Avoiding eye contact to avoid someone talking to you.
- Over-preparing for a talk so that there is absolutely no room for criticism or negative feedback.
- Relying on scripts or running a conversation in your head in details before you take part in it.
- Always organizing for a close friend or family member to be by your side when you attend social occasions.
- Consuming alcohol or substances as a way to numb your fears.
- Changing the way you dress to avoid being noticed.
- Asking someone else too many questions so you don't have to talk about yourself.
- Styling your hair in a way that hides your face if you fear blushing.
- Trying to please everyone all the time to avoid rejection or criticism.

Tip Two: Don't feel like you have to get rid of all your anxiety in these situations. Remember the lessons learned from mindfulness practice. It is okay to feel emotions like worry or embarrassment. Instead of fighting them, allow them to "be" and carry on with your goal for the day.

Tip Three: If you try out exposure therapy and some exercises are a "flop," try to maintain a sense of humor around what happened and if possible, use "failure" for further growth. For instance, if you called someone about the homework but got flustered and you hung up the phone, the next time, you might simply tell them that you forgot what you had to say and that would call back when you remembered.

PRACTICAL EXAMPLES OF EXPOSURE
THERAPY AT WORK

Conquering the Fear of Social Situations

Build a strategy when you tackle your list of anxiety-causing situations. Break down a big goal (such as inviting someone to do something over the weekend) into smaller ones. Start with easy scenarios and add an element of difficulty as you go along. Your list of steps might look something like this:[4]

1. I will ask someone at school what the date is.
2. When I'm seated in the school bus, I will say a couple of things to the person next to me. I might say something about the weather or comment on the bumpy roads.
3. I will give someone a compliment today.
4. I will talk to a classmate I like and have conversed with before.
5. I will approach a group that is chatting and try to join their conversation.
6. I will express my viewpoint during class discussion.
7. I will call a classmate.
8. I will ask someone to come over to study.
9. I will suggest we do something fun on the weekend.
10. I will join a plan that involves being in a group.
11. I will throw a small dinner party at home and invite someone I like but don't know too well.

Conquering the Fear of Presenting a Project to Your Class at School

Oral assessment is common in many schools and colleges, but even if you don't have to face an oral exam, you may be asked to present a project before your classmates and answer their questions. This can be very challenging if your social anxiety involves a fear of speaking in public or being the center of attention. Break this task up as follows:

1. Prepare cards containing the main points you wish to mention about your project. Avoid writing a whole script, since you could end up reading it instead of addressing your classmates. For your speech to be effective, it is important to look at others and use hand gestures to emphasize important parts of your presentation.

2. Practice your presentation in front of a trusted adult (such as a parent, sibling, or good friend).

3. Ask the person assisting you to interrupt you when they need clarification, or when they want to ask a question.

4. Join a theater group at your school, asking for a small role to begin with.

5. Let a group of trusted classmates know you are a little anxious before you start, so they can support you, ease your worries, and make sure to ask questions you are confident about answering.

Conquering the Fear of Eating in Public

Feelings of anxiety about eating in public can stem from several causes. For instance, you may only fear eating in the company of people you don't know well, or you may usually avoid eating in crowded restaurants or attending a formal dinner party. Sometimes, anxiety can be centered on specific food items. For instance, you might find it bearable to eat finger foods in public, but dread consuming soup or noodles. You may fear that you will spill food, your hands will shake, or you will choke. If you have a fear of eating in public, the following activities may be of help:

1. Go to a small restaurant with a good friend or family member at an off-peak time and order something you find easy to eat—for instance, french fries and a drink.
2. Go to a restaurant at a standard meal time with the same person and order two items.
3. Go to lunch with your classmates and order items you are comfortable with.
4. Buy a ticket to a fundraising dinner for yourself and a friend or family member and try to enjoy at least a few bites of every dish.
5. Join your volunteer group for a burger or quick bite after a day out cleaning the park or beach.

6. Book a table at a busy restaurant and challenge yourself with a starter you find a little difficult to eat (such as soup). Go with a friend and, eventually, invite more people.

Conquering the Fear of Dating

If you are an older teen, you may be interested in getting to know someone you are interested in. However, the more they matter to you or the more interested you are, the more anxiety can get in the way of getting to know them. You can take it a little at a time by setting yourself the following goals:

1. Go up to someone you like and ask them how they are doing.
2. Try to extend the amount of time you spend chatting, so you can find out the things they are interested in. If you share an interest, ask them for their number so you can send them information, a sound bite, or video they might like.
3. Call them one weekend and mention something funny you just learned about the band/influencer/channel you both like.
4. Attend a party you know they will be at.

5. Ask them to join you to a concert/film/festival you think you will both enjoy.

Conquering the Fear of Starting, Joining, and Ending Conversations

Forming part of a conversation can be very challenging for teens as a whole, because they may not have the experience required to know when the timing is right. They may also end conversations abruptly. Research by UCLA scientists has shown that spending time on digital devices is no help, since it can interfere with your ability to read others' emotions.[5] Face-to-face communication is, essentially, a much better teacher of how to read emotional cues than texts or verbal calls.

A 2018 study, meanwhile, has shown that teens can find it hard to differentiate between emotions when someone is speaking—a problem that adults do not generally have.[6] For instance, they can find it harder to read emotions such as anger, happiness, or disgust, in their peers. The researchers added that this issue disappears as teens' brains develop and they gain vital life experience.

Experience is a great teacher, but you are never too young to learn a few handy conversational tips.

1. To start a conversation, first, try to work out if it's the right time to do so. If you approach someone and they say hello or smile at you and seem unoccupied, you can use a conversation starter such as, "How are you doing today?" "What are you up to?" "How was class?" or similar. Asking questions is always a great way to get a conversation started, because people often enjoy talking about their interests and the things that are going on in their lives. Another starter involves asking for information, help, or someone's opinion. Take note of the person's body language before starting a conversation. If they are looking away, turning their body away from you, or busy writing a text, it might be better to try when they are freer or in a conversational mood.

2. To join a conversation, first observe the group of people talking. If they are relaxed and engaged in lively conversation, approach them and ask, "Can I join you?" Listen to what they are talking about and show your interest by saying things like, "Wow, that's amazing!" or "That sounds cool." Asking a few questions can also show that you are interested. If, on the other hand, they seem to be discussing

something serious, or they are huddled and have their backs turned to you, it might not be the best time to join in.

3. To end a conversation, be careful of other person's feelings. Try to avoid announcing you'll leave when they are mid-thought or mid-sentence. Thank them and let them know you have to go. Just a few phrases that may come in handy include: "Thanks for that chat. I have to go to class now, but let's talk soon!" "My ride is waiting for me. I have to go. It was great catching up with you!" or "I'd love to hear more about your Chinese language lessons. I have to go now but I hope to learn more about it next time. Have a great afternoon."

You can also break up these tasks into smaller steps. For instance, you might begin by approaching someone you like and are comfortable with in class, then approach a new student or someone you don't know too well. Finally, you might challenge yourself by joining a big group in conversation.

DOCUMENTING YOUR EXPERIENCES

Use your journal to document how you felt when you confronted your fears. This will serve to track your progress and boost your self-confidence, since every fear conquered can help you grow in confidence. Write down what happened, the moments during which you felt most distressed, and new strategies you might try next time. Rate your distress from one to ten. Keep practicing the exposure exercise, journaling your results until your distress ratings go down to half what they originally were.[7]

Exposure therapy, which is a type of cognitive-behavioral therapy, is one of the most challenging yet effective strategies to help you overcome social anxiety. It is usually undertaken with the help of a therapist, who can work alongside you to create your list of stressful situations and suggest ways that you can brave them. If a therapist is not accessible to you, you can try a few techniques out. This will take work and reflection, but "pushing yourself" into challenging situations is one of the few ways to see, with your own eyes, that many of the things you fear never happen at all. Moreover, even if they do happen, they probably won't have a huge impact on your life as a whole.

One of the best features of exposure therapy is that you can take it step by step, exposing yourself to low-anxiety situations before tackling high-stress ones. Keep a journal, so you can see the strategies and phrases that work best for you. Take note of your progress and congratulate yourself on every goal achieved, as well as on the effort you are making to enjoy conversations and build meaningful relationships with others.

8

I AM LOOKING AFTER MYSELF

66 *"When you say "yes" to others make sure you are
not saying "no" to yourself."*

— PAULO COELHO

I n previous chapters, we provided you with
information that will help you understand more
about SAD. We also suggested various exercises you
might like to try out. All of this requires effort, work,
and consistency. However, we have saved the best for
last—self-care. We previously touched on self-kindness
and its ability to reduce stress and to combat issues
such as perfectionism. Looking after yourself is a
holistic pursuit; it involves working on your body and
mind, so you can brave challenges with energy, motiva-

tion, and a positive mentality. Doing so is very difficult if you are tired, burned out, or fatigued.

MAKING THE MOST OF THE MIND-BODY CONNECTION

It is difficult to be happy if your physical health and wellbeing are compromised. It is also hard to feel strong and function at your best physically if your mental health and wellbeing are compromised. Psychoneuroimmunology is the study of the connection between the brain, the emotions, the central nervous system, and the immune system. It espouses that psychological stress can make you more susceptible to everything from colds and the flu, right through to autoimmune disease.[1]

Stress can make your body react as though it was battling an infection or another physical illness. It prompts the brain to produce cytokines—small proteins that help control the growth and activity of immune cells. When you are chronically stressed, your brain produces cytokines over a sustained period. Cytokines are inflammatory—they increase the likelihood of developing a host of physical diseases, including Type II diabetes, heart disease, osteoporosis, allergies, and autoimmune diseases.

STRESS CAN HARM YOU IN THE LONG-TERM

For an idea of how stress and traumatic experiences can affect your health in the future, check out research published by the Association for Psychological Science.[2] The study showed that bullying in childhood can lead to serious illness, difficulties with holding down a job, and poor social relationships when you are an adult. Bullying is not a harmless or inevitable part of maturing and putting up with stress stoically can also cause damage. Consider stress as an inevitable part of life, but one you need to keep in check proactively on a daily basis.

"SITTING" WITH YOUR EMOTIONS

When discussing mindfulness, we mentioned the importance of accepting your emotions instead of repressing them. Accept both good and bad emotions, checking in with them during quiet moments of your day. The following exercise, which involves simply "being" with your emotions, can help you feel more empowered:[3]

1. Sit in a comfortable spot and start by doing a little belly breathing (for around three to five minutes).

2. Let your mind go to a recent situation that you found stressful.

3. Try to identify the emotions you felt at the time, using Plutchik's Wheel of Emotions (which we mentioned in Chapter Three).

4. Scan your body and try noticing how it responds to stress. For instance, you may feel a specific part of your body tense up, or notice that you clench your fists or press your chest with your fingers.

5. Stay with your emotions and sensations. If your mind wanders, come back to the place where you have a bodily sensation that indicates stress. Ride out the sensations, allowing them to exist until they subside.

6. Be aware of any images or memories that pop up in mind.

7. Stay as long as you need to, ending the exercise you feel your emotions are more regulated.

8. Slowly open your eyes and notice how you feel.

STAYING PHYSICALLY ACTIVE

Numerous studies have shown that exercise is a power natural stress and anxiety buster. It lowers levels of the stress hormone, cortisol; lifts the mood; and helps you feel more energetic. By contrast, a lack of physical activity is linked to increased symptoms of anxiety and depression. Exercise can help by:[4]

- Immersing you in the joy of the activity itself, so you can keep your mind "in the present moment."
- Decreasing muscle tension through body movement.
- Increasing your heart rate and promoting positive changes in your brain chemistry. Physical activity boosts the availability of feel-good neurochemicals like serotonin and GABA.
- Activating the frontal regions of the brain, which help keep the amygdala in check.
- Building your resilience, so you can stand up to stress more efficiently.

Why Exercise is Particularly Important if You Have Social Anxiety

If you want to embrace a powerful, cost-effective way to prevent and reduce the symptoms of SAD, get active.

Working out is something that anyone can do, regardless of their age. One 2021 study found that a high intensity exercise regimen (comprising two one-hour swim sessions per week, one weekly hour-long session of indoor sport, and one weekly hour-long session of outdoor sports) was a promising means to quell social anxiety.[5] Another study showed that people with SAD benefited from a combination of physical activity and group cognitive-behavioral therapy.[6]

Motivating Yourself to Exercise

Workouts are one thing that are easy to give up and very hard to restart after a long pause. Even though you know how great you feel after a hard exercise session or run and a shower, it can be hard to get back into the swing of things. These tips will help you feel more like pushing your body to new limits.

- **Start small.** If you haven't been to the gym in a while, starting out with a one-hour workout may leave you sore and unwilling to return the next day. Commence with a 15-minute walk and regularly build up your speed and total workout time. When you start feeling more confident, consider signing up for a class you think you might enjoy—like spin cycling, CrossFit, or hip-hop dancing.

- **Try a group class.** In the previous chapter, we talked about the importance of pushing yourself and saying yes to new challenges. Why not challenge yourself by committing to exercise in a small group? A study published in the *Journal of Social Sciences* showed that people gravitate towards the exercise behaviors of those around them.[7] Therefore, if the people in your group regularly make it to the gym or head to the mountains for a trek, you may be more likely to remain at their level.

- **Go high-intensity.** Exercise at any level can help you eliminate tension, but if you can, ensure at least some of your exercise are high-intensity. A study by University of Missouri-Columbia researchers has found that this type of exercise is more effective at reducing stress and anxiety.[8]

Nobody can really tell you what motivates you to be physically active. Some people enjoy going for a jog alone while listening to ideal running music; others prefer to be joined by a best friend. Be open when it comes to choosing your workout activities and try out new ones. You never know when you might find a new class that is particularly fun or uplifting.

GETTING QUALITY SLEEP

Teens should aim to get between eight and ten hours of sleep every twenty-four hours. Good sleep is not just about quantity, though, it is also about quality. For instance, it is possible to be in bed for ten hours but still wake up sluggish, tired, and with "brain fog."

What Is Good Sleep Quality?

According to The Sleep Foundation, getting good sleep quality involves:

1. Falling asleep quickly once you get into bed (taking a maximum of around 30 minutes to do so).
2. Haven fallen asleep, waking up no more than once per night.
3. Falling back asleep within 20 minutes when you wake up in the middle of the night.
4. Feeling refreshed and energized when you get out of bed in the morning.
5. Getting the recommended number of hours for your age group.

How To Improve Your Sleep Quality

For many people, simply creating a good nighttime routine is enough to put an end to the problem of poor quality sleep. Try these ideas to enjoy a better night's rest:[9]

- **Avoid watching TV or using screen devices for at least half an hour before you sleep.** These devices contain blue light, which your brain perceives as sunlight. This "trick" delays the sensation of sleepiness, since it makes you feel alert.
- **Design a sleep-friendly bedroom.** Invest in blackout curtains (since absolute darkness boosts sleepiness), soundproof your room if you are exposed to sounds at night, and set your thermostat between the low- and mid-60° Fahrenheit, since cool temperatures help you feel sleepier. Make sure your mattress is the right firmness for your sleeping position. For instance, people who sleep on their backs usually benefit from a medium-firm or firm mattress, while those who sleep on their side may favor a medium-soft or medium-firm mattress. Those who sleep on their front may sleep better in a medium or medium-firm mattress.
- **Sleep at the same time every night and follow a relatively strict routine.** For instance, you might take a bath then do a little mindfulness

meditation or progressive muscle relaxation exercises (which we will explain below) before getting into bed.

- **Avoid drinking coffee and other caffeinated drinks in the five hours leading up to your bedtime.**
- **When you wake up, get some sunlight for fifteen minutes minimum.** This will reset your circadian rhythm (the natural process that governs the sleep–wake cycle and repeats every 24 hours).

Using Progressive Muscle Relaxation to Initiate Calm

One ideal exercise to perform right before you sleep is Progressive Muscle Relaxation. This exercise reduces anxiety by making you aware of how difficult emotions manifest themselves through tension in the body. When practiced regularly, it can help you conquer your sleep issues and relieve tension, anxiety, and anger.[10] To perform this technique, follow the steps below:

1. Sit or lie down, taking a few minutes to breathe deeply and relax your body.
2. Tense and relax all your muscles, then let them go. Start with the toes, curling them inwards, pausing, then letting them go. Tense and relax

the muscles in other areas like your knees, thighs, hands, arms, buttocks, and chest (inhaling as you tighten your chest muscles).

3. Raise your shoulders upwards, hold the pose, then release the tension.
4. Open your mouth as widely as you can, pausing, then letting go.
5. Close your eyes as tightly as you can, holding the tension then letting go.
6. Raise your eyebrows, pausing, then letting go.

Progressive Muscle Relaxation has many documented benefits, but for those with anxiety, one of its most useful aspects is that it shows you what parts of your body experience the most tension when you are anxious. It teaches you to be in tune to the connection between your mind and body.

BATTLING SOCIAL ANXIETY THROUGH YOUR DIET

There is a powerful connection between the mind and gut. Researchers have found, for instance, that people with depression have lower levels of specific health-boosting gut bacteria. To ensure you have a wide variety of healthy bacteria in your gut, consume fiber-rich foods, which help gut bacteria thrive.

One study published in the journal, *Diet and Anxiety*, showed that there are dietary patterns that are linked to more or less anxiety.[11]

Foods associated with less anxiety include:

- Fruits and vegetables
- Foods containing Omega-3 essential fatty acids (found in fatty fish like salmon and tuna, extra-virgin olive oil, and walnuts), Omega-9 fatty acids (found in olive oil, avocado oil, and walnuts), and alpha-lipoic acid (sourced from red meat, spinach, carrots, beets, and potatoes).
- Nuts and seeds.
- Foods with *lactobacillus* and *bifidobacterium* (usually found in healthy yogurt varieties).
- Culinary herbs, turmeric, saffron, green tea, and other foods containing antioxidants.

Habits associated with less anxiety include:

- Following the Mediterranean diet (including fruits and vegetables, legumes, and nuts).
- Having breakfast.
- Embracing a vegan lifestyle.
- Consuming vitamins and minerals like Zinc, Selenium, Magnesium, Vitamins C and E, and Choline.

- Following dietary regimens that are not high in carbohydrates or calories.

Foods associated with more anxiety include:

- High-fat, high-cholesterol, high trans fat foods. High-cholesterol foods include fatty meat and processed meat such as sausages, animal fats, and full-fat dairy products. Trans fats can be found in commercial baked goods, shortening, microwave popcorn, frozen pizza, fried foods, non-dairy coffee creamer, and stick margarine.
- Low-protein foods.
- High-sugar foods and those with refined carbohydrates (like cookies, cakes, and many refined snacks).

Habits associated with more anxiety include:

- Frequent snacking.
- Failing to consume enough tryptophan (an amino acid that is present in most protein-rich foods—including oats, milk, yogurt, red meat, eggs, fish, and poultry). Tryptophan cannot be synthesized by humans, so you need to source it from food. It is necessary for the maintenance of the body's proteins, muscles, enzymes, and

neurotransmitters. It is also used to make melatonin, which regulates the sleep-wake cycle.[12]

Nutritional Tip: If you love fermented foods like miso, kimchi, sauerkraut, tempeh, or cultured milk and yogurt, take note—they could help you curb your anxiety.[13] Your gut bacteria love fermented foods and, as you know, it is important to help healthful gut bacteria populations thrive if you want to boost your mental health.

FEELING THE POWER OF NATURE

Nature is an incredibly powerful stress buster, with Cornell University researchers finding that just 10 minutes in a natural setting (such as a park, forest, or beach) can make you happier and lessen the effects of physical and mental stress.[14] Another study by researchers at the Max Planck Institute for Human Development found that after an hour-long walk in nature, stress-related brain activity is reduced.[15] The amygdala is less activated in stressful times in people who live in the country, as opposed to those who live in the city. In the study, researchers divided participants into two groups. One took an hour-long walk in the city of Berlin, and another spent the same time walking in the Grunewald forest. The results showed that activity in the amygdala decreased only among those who had walked in nature.

An Activity to Try: Forest Bathing

Forest bathing involves visiting a forest and opening all your senses to the surrounding beauty. When you enter a forest, feast your eyes on the beautiful trees, plants, and flowers around you. Listen to the birds, insects, and wildlife as they move through their majestic home. Gently touch the bark of the trees around you and run your fingers along the smooth surface of leaves. Smell the freshness of wild-growing plants and flowers. If you live in an area with edible berries or other fruits and foraging is permitted in your area, take a few fruits that you can enjoy at home. Always ask the help of someone who knows about forest species first, to ensure that what you are eating is safe and delicious.

Fun Fact: Researchers in Japan have found that trees release compounds called phytoncides, which have antibacterial properties and which explain why "forest bathing" is so beneficial to human health.[16] This activity is easy, fun, and free. It is also deeply relaxing and re-energizing all at once.

Think of stress-prevention strategies as a pillar of keeping your social anxiety in check. The more active one's amygdala is and the greater the divide between the body and mind is, the more likely you are to struggle in social situations. Healing yourself through exercise, a healthy diet, good sleep, and nature experiences will help you be your calmest self, even in the toughest of situations.

PASS IT ON!

You know only too well what it's like to live with social anxiety... and now you have the power to make somebody else's life that little bit easier... Head over to Amazon and tell other readers what you liked about this book and how it helped you – even just a sentence or two could make the world of difference to another teenager.

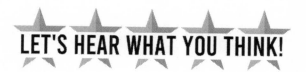

Thank you for being part of the mission to tackle anxiety head-on. I can't tell you how much I appreciate your support, and I truly hope everything you've learned here will help you for a lifetime.

Scan the QR code to leave your review.

CONCLUSION

> ❝ *"The thing that is really hard, and really amazing, is giving up on being perfect and beginning the work of becoming yourself."*
>
> — ANNA QUINDLEN

The teenage years are some of the most memorable in life, but they can also be challenging. The maturing teen brain struggles to adapt to so many demands—such as making and pleasing peers, doing well at school, getting on with authority figures, and excelling at extracurricular activities. During this time, major changes are taking place in your brain, and you are experiencing a huge rise in sex, adrenal, and growth hormone levels. It can be harder to control impulses, which can make social occasions more awkward. Social anxiety can be an additional obstacle, but it is one you can negotiate much more successfully when you learn key strategies.

At the beginning of this book, we delved into the subject of social anxiety and how it differs from typical anxiety. When you have SAD, you dread situations in which you may be judged, or in which you may be the center of attention. Sometimes, your fears can be so vivid and intense that it leads you to avoid social occasions such as parties, lunch dates, and group activities. However, at school, it is often difficult to avoid interacting with others because you may be called upon to work in a group, and simply being in class involves being with other people and sharing information.

If your SAD started to really make its presence felt once you hit your teen years, know that this is typical. Teens have many pressures that children don't, which is why social anxiety manifests itself more intensely during adolescence. Building and maintaining good social relationships are an important buffer against stress, but for someone with social anxiety, being in the presence of others can actually be a cause of anguish.

Throughout the book, we have suggested exercises that are used in cognitive behavioral and dialectical behavior therapies. These exercises can help by teaching you to reframe negative thoughts and beliefs, or take the road of mindful acceptance—recognizing and allowing all thoughts and emotions to exist (including negative ones). Through mindfulness, you can discover that thoughts and feelings are not permanent. They do not define who you are. They can change from moment to moment, even though some of them may persist for a little longer than usual. Thoughts and emotions are like waves that exist in a specific moment. Even though some can seem high, strong, and persistent, they, too, will pass.

Sometimes, social anxiety can lead you into a panicky state. This is when controlled breathing will be your best ally. One of the most amazing things about controlled breathing is how quickly it makes a difference. A few seconds into belly breathing, for instance, you may notice your heart rate drop as your body begins to understand that it isn't actually in a fight or flight situation.

The road to overcoming social anxiety begins by knowing what you're up against. Be aware of destructive habits such as using mental filters, engaging in all-or-nothing thinking, or assuming what others think of you. These irrational thoughts can erode your self-esteem and stop you from taking part in many of the activities you would love to try. Remember that these thoughts are not actually true. They are the result of social anxiety trying to "play a trick" on you. You have many powerful tools that will enable you to stop repetitive thoughts in their tracks—including journaling to reframe negative thoughts into more positive ones.

From the start, working on building strong self-esteem is vital. Doing so will stop you from worrying so much about what others may be thinking. For many people, building good self-esteem is one of the most difficult lifelong tasks they may face. Your self-esteem arises from a myriad of circumstances and experiences, and it can be tough to challenge your self-critic. Do so daily, however, finding things that make you feel better about yourself. Practice daily mindfulness exercises, which will teach you to simply "be" in the present moment instead of worrying about what someone might say.

Building resilience is also important, and the good news is that there are so many ways you can do so. Start by being as kind to yourself as you would to others. Next, sharpen your emotional awareness. Being in tune with how you think and feel is essential, as you can curb negative thoughts quickly before they take over. Other important ways to become stronger include learning how to set boundaries, reminding yourself to put things in perspective, being empathetic to others, and working to achieve your daily and long-term goals.

Remember that your brain is awesome! When you adopt a growth mindset, you realize that everyone is capable of learning new skills and talents. You can be shy at a party today, but decide to go up to a new group at a party tomorrow, practicing a few conversation starters. Who you are today is not who you will be tomorrow. Thanks to neuroplasticity, your brain will continue to grow and change, even when you are in your senior years! Challenge your brain by learning a myriad of new skills like juggling or mastering daily TikTok choreographies.

When you feel overwhelmed, try one of the five grounding techniques we taught you in Chapter Five. These include the 5-4-3-2-1 technique, body awareness, mental exercises, categories, and journaling. Keeping a journal is actually a great way to keep tabs on your biggest challenges and to see how far you are progressing. The more entries you have in your journal, the more you will notice certain patterns that you can work on and the easier it will be to identify the strategies that work for you.

When you feel more resilient, you can try exposure therapy, which involves facing situations that make you feel tense, little by little. This is one of the toughest, yet arguably one of the most effective exercises you will find in this book. Martin Luther King once said, "Our very survival depends on our ability to stay awake, to adjust to new ideas, to remain vigilant and to face the challenge of change."

Finally, look after yourself. Exercise, rest, good nutrition, and spending time in nature can all restore your energy levels and help you feel strong enough to start working on yourself. Remember that conquering social anxiety is not about ending fear (since we all have fears). It is about forging ahead anyway, knowing that even if the very worst thing that could happen occurred, it probably wouldn't matter much a year or two down the track.

We hope you have inspired you to try out various exercises that will help you feel more in control of your social experiences. You will probably find that some strategies work better for you than others. This is to be expected, since we are all individuals and we all use the strategies that resonate with our way of thinking and feeling. Your journal will undoubtedly help you figure out your list of preferred strategies pretty quickly!

If you found this book helpful, we would love it if you could leave us a review on Amazon. Our mission at Succeed Now is to support teens and young adults who are battling social anxiety and other anxiety-related disorders, and we hope the information we share reaches as wide an audience as possible. If even one exercise, thought, or idea helps readers understand they are more powerful even than the most intense feelings of anxiety, then we will have achieved our goal. Thank you for reading!

NOTES

INTRODUCTION

1. Evolve Treatment Centers, n.d.
2. U.S. Department of Health & Human Services, n.d.
3. Massabrook, 2022.
4. Fun With Kids in LA, n.d.

1. I AM BEATING ANXIETY

1. Cleveland Clinic, 2019.
2. Mayo Clinic, n.d.
3. Bridges to Recovery, n.d.
4. Strum, 2022.
5. Morin, 2022.
6. Paradigm Treatment, n.d.
7. Stonewater Adolescent Recovery Center, n.d.
8. Leuker & van den Bos, 2016.
9. Prnicing, 2021.
10. Meuret et al., 2010.
11. Clark, n.d.
12. Healthline, 2019.

2. I AM IN THE PRESENT

1. Cuncic, 2021.
2. Ackerman, 2017.
3. Kuru et al., 2018.
4. Burns, 2000.
5. Grinspoon, 2022.

6. Cuncic, 2020.
7. Raes et al., 2013.
8. Björling et al., 2019.
9. Huppert & Johnson, 2010.
10. Riegner et al., 2022.
11. Kids Health, n.d.
12. Edgar Snyder, n.d.

3. I AM RESILIENT

1. Ko & Chang, 2018.
2. Swayne, 2015.
3. Ferrari, 2018.
4. Moore, 2019.
5. Six Seconds, n.d.
6. Crime Victim Center of Erie County, n.d.
7. Cherry, 2022.
8. Truity, n.d.
9. Beaton, 2017.
10. Anderson & Jiang, 2018.
11. Raising Children, n.d.

4. I HAVE A STRONG MINDSET

1. Cullins, 2022.
2. Mayfield Clinic, n.d.
3. Metivier, 2022.
4. Gage, 2022.
5. Cherry, 2022.
6. Teh, 2021.
7. Dweck, 2006.
8. Weiss, 2020.
9. Cullins, 2022.
10. WDHB, 2021.

5. I CAN MANAGE MY EMOTIONS

1. Cleveland Clinic, n.d.
2. Dodson, 2022.
3. Goldin et al., 2009.
4. Dixon et al., 2020.
5. Davis, n.d.
6. Therapist Aid, n.d.
7. Shaarawy, 2014.
8. Boogaard, 2020.
9. Smyth et al., 2018.
10. Ghavami, 2022.
11. Scott, 2021.

6. I CAN QUESTION MYSELF

1. Leadem, 2017.
2. Abraham, 2020.
3. Williams, 2017.
4. Inner Melbourne Clinical Psychology, n.d.
5. Gosnell, 2019.
6. Benoliel, 2017.
7. Davila & Beck, 2022.
8. HelpGuide, n.d.
9. Healthy WA, n.d.
10. Trew & Alden, 2015.

7. I CAN PUSH MYSELF

1. Lim, 2016.
2. Mayo Clinic, n.d.
3. Chand, 2019.
4. Cuncic, 2021.
5. Wolpert, 2014.
6. Morningstar et al., 2018.

7. Therapist Aid, n.d.

8. I AM LOOKING AFTER MYSELF

1. Choix, n.d.
2. Wolke et al., 2013.
3. Choix, n.d.
4. Ratey, 2019..
5. Zika & Becker, 2021.
6. Merom et al., 2008.
7. Steinhilber, 2017.
8. Science Daily, 2003.
9. Sleep Foundation, 2022.
10. de Lorent et al., 2016.
11. Aucoin et al., 2021.
12. MedlinePlus, n.d.
13. Aslam et al., 2020.
14. Meredith et al., 2020.
15. Sudimac et al., 2022.
16. Science Daily, 2018.

REFERENCES

Abraham, M. (2020, October 10). *Anxiety and irrational thoughts.* CalmClinic. https://www.calmclinic.com/anxiety/signs/crazy-thoughts

Ackerman, C. E. (2017, September 29). *Cognitive distortions: 22 examples & worksheets (& PDF).* https://positivepsychology.com/cognitive-distortions/

Anderson, M., & Jiang, J. (2018, November 28). *Teens, friendships and online groups.* Pew Research Center. https://www.pewresearch.org/internet/2018/11/28/teens-friendships-and-online-groups/

Aslam, H., Green, J., Jacka, F. N., Collier, F., Berk, M., Pasco, J., & Dawson, S. L. (2020, September 23). Fermented foods, the gut and mental health: a mechanistic overview with implications for depression and anxiety. *Nutritional Neuroscience, 23*(9), 659-671. https://doi.org/10.1080/1028415X.2018.1544332

Aucoin, M., LaChance, L., Naidoo, U., Remy, D., Shekdar, T., Sayar, N., Cardozo, V., Rawana, T., Chan, I., & Cooley, K. (2021, December 13). Diet and anxiety: A scoping review. *Nutrients, 13*(12). https://doi.org/10.3390/nu13124418

Beaton, C. (2017, October 6). *The majority of people are not introverts or extroverts.* Psychology Today. https://www.psychologytoday.com/us/blog/the-gen-y-guide/201710/the-majority-people-are-not-introverts-or-extroverts

Benoliel, B. (2017, May 30). *What's your conflict management style?* Walden University. https://www.waldenu.edu/news-and-events/walden-news/2017/0530-whats-your-conflict-management-style

Björling, E. A., Stevens, C., Sing, N. B. (2019, May 22). Participatory pilot of an art-based mindfulness intervention for adolescent girls with headache. *Art Therapy, 36*(2), 86-92. https://doi.org/10.1080/07421656.2019.1609325

Boogaard, K. (2020, March 26). *Why you need to start using a decision journal.* Trello. https://blog.trello.com/decision-journal

Bridges to Recovery. (n.d.). *Causes of social anxiety.* https://www. bridgestorecovery.com/social-anxiety/causes-social-anxiety/

Burns, D. D. (2000). *Feeling good* (2nd ed.). Harper.

Chand, S. (2019, November 23). *Social anxiety: Beware the silken trap of safety behaviors.* National Social Anxiety Center. https://nationalso cialanxietycenter.com/2019/11/23/social-anxiety-beware-the-silken-trap-of-safety-behaviors/

Cherry, K. (2022, August 4). *What are the big 5 personality traits?* Verywell Mind. https://www.verywellmind.com/the-big-five-personal ity-dimensions-2795422

Cherry, K. (2022, September 19). *What is neuroplasticity?* Verywell Mind. https://www.verywellmind.com/what-is-brain-plasticity-2794886

Choix, J. (n.d.). *The mind-body connection and anxiety.* MyWellbeing. https://mywellbeing.com/workplace-wellbeing/mind-body-connection

Clark, B. (n.d.). *Are you a belly breather or a chest breather? Does it matter?* Yoga International. https://yogainternational.com/article/view/are-you-a-belly-breather-or-a-chest-breather-does-it-matter

Cleveland Clinic. (2019, December 9). *What happens to your body during the fight or flight response?* https://health.clevelandclinic.org/what-happens-to-your-body-during-the-fight-or-flight-response/

Cleveland Clinic. (n.d.). *Emotional stress: Warning signs, management, when to get help.* https://my.clevelandclinic.org/health/articles/6406-emotional-stress-warning-signs-management-when-to-get-help

Crime Victim Center of Erie County. (n.d.). *Healthy boundaries for teens.* https://cvcerie.org/healthy-boundaries-for-teens/

Cullins, A. (2022, June 23). *Fixed mindset vs. growth mindset quiz.* Big Life Journal. https://biglifejournal.com/blogs/blog/fixed-mindset-vs-growth-mindset-quiz

Cullins, A. (2022, August 23). *How to explain growth mindset to kids:*

Neuroplasticity activities. Big Life Journal. https://biglifejournal.com/blogs/blog/teach-kids-growth-mindset-neuroplasticity-activities

Cuncic, A. (2020, March 21). *How self-esteem affects social anxiety disorder.* Verywell Mind. https://www.verywellmind.com/self-esteem-and-social-anxiety-4158220

Cuncic, A. (2021, March 27). *How do I get over my fear of social situations?* Verywell Mind. https://www.verywellmind.com/how-do-i-get-over-my-fear-of-social-situations-3024829

Cuncic, A. (2021, October 11). *Overcome negative thinking when you have social anxiety disorder.* Verywell Mind. https://www.verywellmind.com/how-to-stop-thinking-negatively-3024830

Davila, J., & Beck, J. G. (Summer, 2022). Is social anxiety associated with impairment in close relationships? A preliminary investigation. *Behavior Therapy, 33*(3), 427-446. https://doi.org/10.1016/S0005-7894(02)80037-5

Davis, T. (n.d.). *What is reappraisal—And how do you do it?* Berkeley Well-Being Institute. https://www.berkeleywellbeing.com/reappraisal.html

de Lorent, L., Agorastos, A., Yassouridis, A., Kellner, M., & Muhtz, C. (2016, August). Auricular acupuncture versus progressive muscle relaxation in patients with anxiety disorders or major depressive disorder: a prospective parallel group clinical trial. *Journal of Acupuncture and Meridian Studies, 9*(4), 191-199. https://doi.org/10.1016/j.jams.2016.03.008.

Dixon, M. L., Moodie, C. A., Goldin, P. R., Farb, N., Heimberg, R. G., & Gross, J. J. (2020, January 1). Emotion regulation in social anxiety disorder: Reappraisal and acceptance of negative self-beliefs. *Biological Psychiatry: Cognitive Neuroscience and Neuroimaging, 5*(1), 119-129. https://doi.org/10.1016/j.bpsc.2019.07.009

Dodson, W. (2022, June 6). *[Self-test] Could you have emotional hyperarousal?* ADDitude. https://www.additudemag.com/emotional-hyperarousal-adhd-self-test/

Dweck, C. S. (2006). *Mindset: The new psychology of success.* Random House.

Edgar Snyder. (n.d.). *Texting and driving accident statistics.* https://www.

edgarsnyder.com/car-accident/cause-of-accident/cell-phone/cell-phone-statistics.html

Evolve Treatment Centers. (n.d.). *Teen stress and anxiety: facts and statistics.* https://evolvetreatment.com/blog/teen-stress-anxiety-facts/

Ferrari M., Yap, K., Scott, N., Einstein, D. A., & Ciarrochi, J. (2018, February 21). Self-compassion moderates the perfectionism and depression link in both adolescence and adulthood. *PLOS ONE, 13*(2). https://doi.org/10.1371/journal.pone.0192022

Fun With Kids in LA. (n.d.). *20 free mental health services and resources for youth and their families!* https://www.funwithkidsinla.com/post/20-free-mental-health-services-and-resources-for-youth-and-their-families

Gage, F. H. (2022, April 1). Structural plasticity of the adult brain. *Dialogues in Clinical Neuroscience, 6*(2), 135-141. https://doi.org/10.31887/DCNS.2004.6.2/fgage

Ghavami, T., Kazemini,a M., & Rajati, F. (2022, April 13). The effect of lavender on stress in individuals: A systematic review and meta-analysis. *Complementary Therapies in Medicine, 68.* https://doi.org/10.1016/j.ctim.2022.102832

Goldin, P. R., Manber, T., Hakimi, S., Canli, T., & Gross, J. J. (2009, February). Neural basis of social anxiety disorder: Emotional reactivity and cognitive regulation during social and physical threat. *Archives of General Psychiatry, 66*(2), 170-180. https://doi.org/10.1001/archgenpsychiatry.2008.525

Gosnell, S. (2019, August 18). *Positive conflict in the workplace.* Exude. https://www.exudeinc.com/blog/positive-conflict-in-the-workplace/

Grinspoon, P. (2022, May 4). *How to recognize and tame your cognitive distortions.* Harvard Health Publishing. https://www.health.harvard.edu/blog/how-to-recognize-and-tame-your-cognitive-distortions-202205042738

Healthline. (2019, April 22). *8 breathing exercises to try when you feel anxious.* https://www.healthline.com/health/breathing-exercises-for-anxiety

Healthy WA. (n.d.). *Assertive communication.* https://www.healthywa.wa. gov.au/Articles/A_E/Assertive-communication

Heggeness, G. (2020, October 12). *24 quotes about helping others.* Pure-Wow. https://www.purewow.com/entertainment/quotes-about-helping-others

HelpGuide. (n.d.). *Conflict resolution skills.* https://www.helpguide.org/ articles/relationships-communication/conflict-resolution-skills.htm

Huppert, F. A., & Johnson, D. M. (2010, August 3). A controlled trial of mindfulness training in schools: The importance of practice for an impact on well-being. The *Journal of Positive Psychology, 5*(4), 264-274. https://doi.org/10.1080/17439761003794148

Inner Melbourne Clinical Psychology. (n.d.). *How thought challenging can help you to curb negative thinking spirals.* https://www.innermelbpsy chology.com.au/thought-challenging/

Kids Health. (n.d.). *Mindfulness exercises.* https://kid-shealth.org/Nemours/en/teens/mindful-exercises.html

Ko, C. A., & Chang, Y. (2018, January 29). Investigating the relation-ships among resilience, social anxiety, and procrastination in a sample of college students. *SAGE Journals, 122*(1), 231-245. https://doi.org/10.1177/0033294118755111

Kuru, E., Safak, Y., Ozdemir, I., Tulaci, R. G., Özdel, K., Özkula, N. G., & Örsel, S. (2018, April–June). Cognitive distortions in patients with social anxiety disorder: Comparison of a clinical group and healthy controls. *European Journal of Psychiatry, 32*(2), 97-104. https://doi: 10.1016/j.ejpsy.2017.08.004

Leadem, R. (2017, November 9). *These artists, authors and leaders battled self-doubt before they made history.* Entrepreneur. https://www. entrepreneur.com/leadership/these-artists-authors-and-leaders-battled-self-doubt/304340

Leuker, C., & van den Bos, W. (2016, June). I want it now! the neuro-science of teenage impulsivity. *Frontiers for Young Minds, 4*(29). https://doi:10.3389/frym.2016.00008

Lim, M. H. (2016, November 24). *Explainer: what is exposure therapy and how can it treat social anxiety?* The Conversation. https://theconversa

tion.com/explainer-what-is-exposure-therapy-and-how-can-it-treat-social-anxiety-64483

Linehan, M. (2022). *Cope ahead skill*. Dialectical Behavior Therapy (DBT) Tools. https://dbt.tools/emotional_regulation/cope-ahead.php

Massabrook, N. (2022, February 27). *Ryan Reynolds says anxiety leaves him feeling like a 'different person' sometimes: 'I have 2 parts of my personality'*. US Magazine. https://www.usmagazine.com/celebrity-news/news/ryan-reynolds-anxiety-leaves-him-feeling-like-a-different-person/

Mayfield Clinic. (n.d.). *Anatomy of the brain*. https://mayfieldclinic.com/pe-anatbrain.htm

Mayo Clinic. (n.d.). *Social anxiety disorder (Social phobia)*. https://www.mayoclinic.org/diseases-conditions/social-anxiety-disorder/symptoms-causes/syc-20353561

Medline Plus. (n.d.). *Tryptophan*. https://medlineplus.gov/ency/article/002332.htm

Meredith, G. R., Rakow, D. A., Eldermire, E. R. B., Madsen, C. G., Shelley, S. P., & Sachs, N. A. (2020, January 14). Minimum time dose in nature to positively impact the mental health of college-aged students, and how to measure it: A scoping review. *Frontiers in Psychology, 10*. https://doi.org/10.3389/fpsyg.2019.02942

Merom, D., Phongsavan, P., Wagner, R., Chey, T., Marnane, C., Steel, Z., Silove, D., & Bauman, A. (2008, August). Promoting walking as an adjunct intervention to group cognitive behavioral therapy for anxiety disorders—A pilot group randomized trial. *Journal of Anxiety Disorders, 22*(6), 959-968. https://doi.org/10.1016/j.janxdis.2007.09.010

Metivier, A. (2022, July 28). *What is prospective memory? Everything you needed to know*. Magnetic Memory Method. https://www.magneticmemorymethod.com/prospective-memory/

Meuret, A. E., Rosenfield, D., Seidel, A., Bhaskara, L., & Hofmann, S. G. (2010). *Journal of Consulting and Clinical Psychology, 78*(5), 691-704. https://doi.org/10.1037/a0019552

Mindful. (n.d.). *How to meditate with anxiety.* https://www.mindful.org/mindfulness-meditation-anxiety/

Moore, C. (2019, June 2). *How to practice self-compassion: 8 techniques and tips.* Positive Psychology. https://positivepsychology.com/how-to-practice-self-compassion/

Morin, A. (2022, September 1). *What is peer pressure?* Verywell Family. https://www.verywellfamily.com/negative-and-positive-peer-pressure-differences-2606643

Morningstar, M., Ly, V. Y., Feldman, L., & Dirks, M. A. (2018, January 16). Mid-adolescents' and adults' recognition of vocal cues of emotion and social intent: Differences by expression and speaker age. *Journal of Nonverbal Behavior, 42,* 237-251. https://link.springer.com/article/10.1007/s10919-018-0274-7

Paradigm Treatment. (n.d.). *Common causes of anxiety in teens and young adults.* https://paradigmtreatment.com/anxiety-teens-young-adults/common-causes/

Princing, M. (2021, September 1). *This is why deep breathing makes you feel so chill.* Right as Rain by UW Medicine. https://rightasrain.uwmedicine.org/mind/stress/why-deep-breathing-makes-you-feel-so-chill

Raes, F., Griffith, J. W., Van der Guvht, K., & Williams, M. G. (2013, March 6). School-based prevention and reduction of depression in adolescents: A cluster-randomized controlled trial of a mindfulness group program. *Mindfulness, 5,* 477-486. https://doi.org/10.1007/s12671-013-0202-1

Raising Children. (n.d.). *Problem-solving steps: pre-teens and teenagers.* https://raisingchildren.net.au/pre-teens/behaviour/encouraging-good-behaviour/problem-solving-steps

Ratey, J. J. (n.d.). *Can exercise help treat anxiety?* Harvard Health Publishing. https://www.health.harvard.edu/blog/can-exercise-help-treat-anxiety-2019102418096

Riegner, G., Posey, G., Oliva, V., Jung, Y., Mobley, W., & Zeidan, F. (2022, July 7). Disentangling self from pain: mindfulness meditation–induced pain relief is driven by thalamic–default mode network decoupling. *PAIN*, *10*. https://doi: 10.1097/j.pain.0000000000002731

Science Daily. (2003, July 15). *High-intensity exercise best way to reduce anxiety, University of Missouri study finds.* https://www.sciencedaily. com/releases/2003/07/030715091511.htm

Science Daily. (2018, July 6). *It's official—Spending time outside is good for you.* https://www.sciencedaily.com/releases/2018/07/ 180706102842.htm

Scott, E. (2021, March 31). *Journaling to cope with anxiety.* Verywell Mind. https://www.verywellmind.com/journaling-a-great-tool-for-coping-with-anxiety-3144672

Shaarawy, H. Y. (2014, October). The effect of journal writing on students' cognitive critical thinking skills a quasi-experiment research on an EFL undergraduate classroom in Egypt. *International Journal of Higher Education, 3*(4), 120-128. https://doi.org/10.5430/ijhe.v3n4p120

Six Seconds. (n.d.). *Plutchik's wheel of emotions: Exploring the emotion wheel.* https://www.6seconds.org/2022/03/13/plutchik-wheel-emotions/

Skurat, K. (2021, November 16). *Tips to deal with emotional overwhelm.* We Heart. https://www.we-heart.com/2021/03/04/seven-tips-to-deal-with-emotional-overwhelm-that-work/

Sleep Foundation. (2022, March 11). *How to determine poor sleep quality.* https://www.sleepfoundation.org/sleep-hygiene/how-to-deter mine-poor-quality-sleep

Smyth, J., Johnson, J. A., Auer, B. J., Lehman, E., Talamo, G., & Scia-manna, C. N. (2018, October–December). *JMIR Mental Health, 5*(4). https://doi.org/10.2196/11290

Steinhilber, B. (2017, September 15). *The health benefits of working out with a crowd.* NBC News. https://www.nbcnews.com/better/ health/why-you-should-work-out-crowd-ncna798936

Stonewater Adolescent Recovery Center. (n.d.). *3 ways hormones impact teen mental health.* https://www.stonewaterrecovery.com/adoles cent-treatment-blog/3-ways-hormones-impact-teen-mental-health/

Strum, J. (2022, May 2). *What age do most teens first use drugs or alcohol?* The Recovery Village. https://www.therecoveryvillage.com/teen-addiction/age-teens-first-use-drugs-and-alcohol/

Sudimac, S., Sale, V., & Kühn, S. (2022, September 5). How nature nurtures: Amygdala activity decreases as the result of a one-hour walk in nature. *Molecular Psychiatry.* https://doi.org/10.1038/s41380-022-01720-6

Swayne, M. (2015, April 23). *Resilience, not abstinence, may help teens battle online risk.* Penn State University. https://www.psu.edu/news/research/story/resilience-not-abstinence-may-help-teens-battle-online-risk/

Teh, C. (2021, August 15). Neuroplasticity and video games. *The Scientific Teen.* https://www.thescientificteen.org/post/neuroplasticity-and-video-games

Therapist Aid. (n.d.). *Exposure tracking log.* https://www.therapistaid.com/therapy-worksheet/exposure-tracking-log

Therapist Aid. (n.d.). *Grounding techniques.* https://www.therapistaid.com/worksheets/grounding-techniques

Trew, J. L., & Alden, L. E. (2015, June 5). Kindness reduces avoidance goals in socially anxious individuals. *Motivation and Emotion 39,* 892-907. https://doi.org/10.1007/s11031-015-9499-5

Truity. (n.d.). *The big five personality test.* https://www.truity.com/test/big-five-personality-test

U.S. Department of Health & Human Services. (n.d.). *What are the five major types of anxiety disorders?* https://www.hhs.gov/answers/mental-health-and-substance-abuse/what-are-the-five-major-types-of-anxiety-disorders/index.html

WDHB. (2021, September 22). *Growth mindset quiz – Is your mindset fixed or growth?* https://wdhb.com/blog/growth-mindset-quiz/

Weiss, R. (2020, February 25). *To overcome social anxiety, mindset matters.* National Social Anxiety Center. https://nationalsocialanxietycenter.com/2020/02/25/to-overcome-social-anxiety-mindset-matters/

Williams, E. (2017, January 15). *14 irrational thoughts everyone with social anxiety has had before.* Elite Daily. https://www.elitedaily.com/well ness/irrational-thoughts-social-anxiety/1748773

Wolke, D., Copeland, W. E., Angold, A., & Costello, E. J. (2013). Impact of Bullying in Childhood on Adult Health, Wealth, Crime, and Social Outcomes. *Psychological Science, 24*(10), 1958–1970. https://doi.org/10.1177/0956797613481608

Wolpert, S. (2014, August 21). *In our digital world, are young people losing the ability to read emotions?* UCLA. https://newsroom.ucla.edu/releases/in-our-digital-world-are-young-people-losing-the-ability-to-read-emotions

Zika, M. A, & Becker, L. (2021, June 11). Physical activity as a treatment for social anxiety in clinical and non-clinical populations: a systematic review and three meta-analyses for different study designs. *Frontiers of Human Neuroscience, 15.* https://doi.org/10.3389/fnhum.2021.653108

ABOUT THE AUTHOR

Succeed Now is the brand behind *Relief from Social Anxiety and Stress for Teens.*

Their work is focused on adolescent mental health, and provides essential information and tools to help teenagers navigate life's challenges and move towards adulthood with confidence.

Succeed Now is a dedicated team of healthcare professionals who are committed to providing knowledge and essential life skills, not only to teenagers, but to parents and caregivers too.

Between them, the team has over 50 years of experience in mental healthcare, and each member has worked with a wide range of patients, including teenagers. They recognize the importance of developing mental health strategies and social skills at a young age, and the impact that doing this has on a person's happiness and success later in life. Their goal is to provide support for young people with their whole lives in mind, using their experience in healthcare to provide advice informed by evidence-based therapies.

Succeed Now was formed in order to provide accessible, use-friendly material to both young people and their caregivers. The brand is driven by passion and a common goal: to assist readers in dealing with any challenges life throws their way, and help them hone the tools they need to protect their mental health no matter what.

Made in the USA
Columbia, SC
08 November 2023